Your Feet Don't Have to Hurt

Also by Suzanne M. Levine, D.P.M.

50 Ways to Ease Foot Pain

My Feet Are Killing Me!

Walk It Off

Your Feet Don't Have to Hurt

*A Woman's Guide to
Lifelong Foot Care*

*Suzanne M. Levine,
D.P.M.*

St. Martin's Press
New York

www.stmartins.com

LIBRARY OF CONGRESS CATALOGING-IN-PUBLICATION DATA

Levine, Suzanne M.
    Your feet don't have to hurt : a woman's guide to lifelong foot care / Suzanne M.
    Levine with Susan Jacoby.—1st U.S. ed.
        p. cm.
    Includes index.
    ISBN 0-312-26276-0
        1. Foot—Care and hygiene—Popular works. 2. Foot—Diseases—Popular
    works. I. Jacoby, Susan. II. Title.
RD563 .L393 2000
617.5'85—dc21   00-024609

First Edition: June 2000

10   9   8   7   6   5   4   3   2   1

To André Leon Talley

A Note to Readers

This book is for informational purposes only. Readers are advised to consult a trained medical professional before acting on any of the information in this book.

Contents

Contents

Illustrations

Acknowledgments

This book would not have been possible without the assistance of many people. I want to thank my coauthor, Susan Jacoby, for her intelligence, enthusiasm, and invaluable assistance.

I am also grateful to Heather Jackson Silverman, my editor at St. Martin's Press, who believed in this topic from the start, and John Murphy, whose wit and personality inspired some of the anecdotes in the book.

I owe special thanks to André Leon Talley, who helped to make beautiful feet fashionable.

Dr. Everett Lauder's patience and support gave me an immeasurable boost during the long period of writing this book.

I am also grateful to Dr. Bruce Bitcover and Dr. Bruce Zappan, two esteemed colleagues who are truly a step ahead.

How to Use This Book

This book is intended as a consumer's guide to medical foot care, self-care, and pampering to make your feet look as good as they will feel.

Part I presents an overview of your feet—their structure and function at rest and in motion, the reasons why so many things can go wrong, the special problems of women's feet, and the normal changes you can expect with aging.

Part II is a guide to just about everything that can cause foot pain, from minor blisters and corns to major tendon and ligament injuries. Each chapter begins with a brief explanation of the medical condition, followed by a list of the most common symptoms. Individual case histories—all of them taken from my own patient files—tell you what to expect when you're being treated by a podiatrist and give you my views on what works and what doesn't. Although the focus of my book is on treatment of foot pain through nonsurgical means, the last chapter in this section is designed to help you ask the right questions if your doctor recommends an operation.

The closing section of each chapter provides a list of tips on prevention and self-care. These are designed to help you avoid some of the most common foot problems—and to get the best possible results from medical treatment by following up with commonsense self-care measures and lifestyle changes.

Part III discusses the connection between foot pain and problems involving the rest of your body—including lower back disorders, arthritis, and diabetes.

Part IV deals with the many lifestyle factors and life choices—from pregnancy to pedicures—that have a major impact on foot health. I've tried to answer the most common questions posed by patients who make widely varying demands on their feet. Whether you're a jogger who wants to know how to run without hurting your feet, a guilty couch potato who needs to get out of the living room and back *on* your feet, a parent wondering whether your child's walk is really normal, or a woman who simply wants to find shoes that are pretty as well as "sensible," you'll find advice geared to your way of life.

Preface

I became a foot doctor because, for much of my life, I had no idea of how to take care of my own feet—or of what it felt like to enjoy the everyday miracle of fluid, pain-free walking.

Because I was born with unusually wide, flat feet, my parents, acting on the prevailing medical opinion of the late fifties and sixties, had me fitted for heavy orthopedic shoes at age two. Throughout my childhood, I was a reluctant, tearful patient at what was then called the Hospital for the Ruptured and Crippled (now the Hospital for Special Surgery) in New York City. "Crippled" is exactly how I thought of myself as I was fitted, year after year, for ugly lace-up brown oxfords that were supposed to lift up my arches and help correct my bowed legs.

I was discouraged, by doctors and by my own embarrassment about those shoes, from participating in school sports, summer camping, and the ballet and tap-dancing lessons enjoyed by other girls my age. I became a sedentary and overweight child, convinced that my feet would always hurt and that I would always be set apart from my peers as a result of the hideous shoes and inactivity that were supposed to help me.

I finally stepped out on my own (my mother couldn't follow

me to college with the oxfords) when I was a student at Columbia University. I decided to study physical therapy, and I began to learn how to care for my feet. There was certainly no mystery about my attraction to rehabilitative medicine as a future career: My activities had been severely restricted as a child, and I could imagine nothing more fulfilling than helping others regain and retain their mobility.

During those college years, I discovered simple exercises—which are still a part of my daily routine—designed to strengthen my weak arches. I became more mobile in every way, walking instead of riding and enjoying a wide variety of activities—dancing was number one on my list—that had been off-limits to me as a child. I learned when to rest, soak, and massage my feet, which did and do tire easily because of the lack of support from my arches. I also began to indulge a pent-up passion for beautiful shoes.

Because I was forced to wear ugly shoes throughout my teen years, I'm in a better position than most podiatrists to empathize with the resistance of many of my women patients when I tell them that they need to switch from flimsy, pointy-toed high heels on the cutting edge of fashion to less extreme, roomier pumps with lower heels. One of the most important things I learned when I began taking care of my feet in college was that it's possible to find flattering, fashionable shoes that also enable you to stand and walk without pain. Your feet *don't* have to suffer for beauty.

Although I solved most of my personal foot problems in college, only when I began working as a physical therapist did I come to appreciate fully the complex wonder of the mobility most of us take for granted. As a young therapist, I was awed by the tenacity and courage of stroke victims, paraplegics, and amputees—many of them Vietnam war veterans recovering from their wounds—who invested their entire minds and bodies in the slow, painful effort to recover the capacity to put one foot in front of the other. In the midseventies, I decided to go back to school to study podiatry, with the goal of becoming a podiatric surgeon. At the time, foot surgery (like all surgery) was almost exclusively a man's world, but I was determined to take part in the process of rehabilitation at a higher level—to learn how actually to repair grievously hurt feet.

At the time, the New York College of Podiatric Medicine had some of the most outstanding foot surgeons in the country on its faculty. I was one of its few female students. (Even today, although many more women have entered the profession, more than 90 percent of podiatric surgeons are men.) That's ironic, in view of the fact that approximately 80 percent of podiatric *patients* are women—for reasons discussed later in this book. The medical and surgical training I received was first-rate, but some of the older professors pointed to me as an example of someone with "bad" feet—an unpleasant echo from my childhood.

I knew—though I didn't have the authority back then to argue with my teachers—that I had rehabilitated my feet through a self-designed, trial-and-error program of physical therapy. And I knew that when I opened my own practice, I would stress the importance of prevention—of stopping pain before it starts—through self-care. Surgery, and other aggressive medical intervention, would be a last resort. Most of us don't have "bad" feet—but most of us do treat our feet badly.

MOVEMENT AS THE CURE FOR FOOT PAIN

As a podiatrist with twenty years of experience, I know that activity—not inactivity—is the solution to problems like the ones that caused me so much pain and humiliation as a little girl. It is now known that simple exercises and lightweight orthotic inserts for ordinary shoes are often the best prescription for children whose foot problems are similar to the ones I had when I was growing up.

Furthermore, sensible exercise is the real remedy for many of the painful conditions that lead adults to declare, "My feet are killing me." Unlike me, most people don't begin to have trouble with their feet until their thirties. As recently as a generation ago, middle age meant a decline in activity: If your feet or your back hurt, the solution was to flop on the couch and rest those aching body parts, leaving the dancing, softball, and bicycling to the young. The very young. That's no longer the case: Regardless of our age, we all want to participate in the same physical pursuits we've always enjoyed. Fit feet literally provide the foundation for that active life.

As a doctor and an *ex*-patient, I'm convinced that there's no good reason why nearly ninety million adult Americans—the number who say their feet hurt them much of the time—should resign themselves to chronic foot pain. A regular self-care routine, which includes everything from exercises to properly fitting shoes, can keep most of us on our active, pain-free feet not only in midlife but for a lifetime.

More than 80 percent of my patients—even if they come hobbling through my door in so much pain that they're blinking back tears—can be restored to full, pain-free mobility through a combination of minor, noninvasive medical procedures, custom-fitted orthotics, and a follow-up at-home routine of therapeutic exercises and outright foot pampering. Those who do need surgery for more serious conditions can usually look forward to being back on their feet, without crutches, within a few days.

Unfortunately, I've treated many patients who have suffered long and needlessly because, terrified by stories of difficult recoveries from foot operations performed with techniques and instruments now as outdated as rotary telephone dials, they put off going to a doctor for months or years. They simply weren't aware of the advances in computer-aided microsurgery, which have not only minimized postoperative pain but also cut recovery time in half during the past decade.

As a doctor, nothing gives me more satisfaction than putting these fears to rest—and seeing men and women restored to full mobility after years of thinking that they would have to live with foot pain forever. Walking across the street near my Manhattan office last week, I was nearly knocked down by a woman running to catch a bus. She stopped to apologize, and I recognized her as a patient whose large, inflamed bunion I had removed surgically only seven weeks earlier. She was wearing a pair of elegant pumps (with, I noticed, the comfortable one-and-a-half-inch heels I'd recommended). The last time I'd seen her, to remove her stitches, she was wearing a surgical shoe and using a cane. "Caroline,"* I said, "I've been wondering why you haven't come in for your postop checkup. But if you can run that fast, you're doing fine." "You know," she replied, "I just realized that I haven't run in years—not even to catch a bus—and now I'm doing it without thinking. I've stopped expecting the pain to come back and hit me without any warning."

While most of us will never need foot surgery, it's vital to maintain, pay attention to, and respect our feet in the same routine way we watch our weight, have our teeth cleaned by a dentist, and correct our vision with contact lenses or glasses. When printed pages and computer screens blur before our eyes, we don't resign ourselves to poor vision and decide to avoid reading. Yet that's exactly what many people do when their feet hurt: They tell themselves that everyone has to live with foot problems, and they grow more sedentary in an effort to avoid the pain.

Others, by contrast, push on with everything from ordinary walking to long-distance running under the theory of "no pain,

*All patients' names have been changed to protect privacy.

no gain." They ignore the throbbing signals from their feet for weeks, months, even years—until, one day, they step out of bed and find themselves in so much anguish that they can't walk or bear to put on a pair of ordinary shoes. Whether the pain is caused by something as complicated and serious as a ruptured tendon or as simple as an ingrown toenail, these men and women will need more medical help and take longer to recover than they would have if they'd paid attention to the early signs of trouble.

Whatever the cause of your foot pain, I have one message: *Your feet don't have to hurt.* If you're over thirty and have been told that foot pain is inevitable with aging, what you've heard is wrong. And that's true whether you're a woman whose feet bear the scars of a lifetime squeezed into poorly fitting shoes, a jogger who has placed too much stress on the lower body through lack of moderation in exercise, or simply someone who's been told you have "bad feet."

As a woman, I practice what I preach as a doctor—and I'm walking proof that anyone can have fit feet for life. One of the most satisfying experiences of my life was a 1986 vacation in the Alaska wilderness, where I joined a hiking group in the Mt. McKinley area. Only two years earlier, after two pregnancies that added more than fifty pounds to my five-foot-four frame, I had started a program of brisk walking in an effort to lose weight. At that point, all I wanted to do was take off the pounds—but as I gradually worked my way up to three miles in under an hour, I began to enjoy the exercise for its own sake. And my feet—my wonderful, working feet that needed just a little help from orthotic inserts in my ordinary athletic shoes—never let me down.

In Alaska, I discovered that I was equal to the physical demands of serious mountain hiking, and I can still recall the intense joy of sitting atop a small peak, basking in the sun and mountain air as other hikers struggled up the grade. To be first up the mountain—to be walking around in mountain country at all—was something utterly unimaginable to the little girl who was told that ballet and volleyball weren't for her because her feet were too weak.

If I can do it, so can you. My program of foot care, outlined in this book, is really a guide to painless movement, whether you want to take a climb in the mountains or a stroll in a park. Like every other body part, our feet do change, and require more attention, as we age. But if you pay attention to what these anatomical marvels are telling you, your feet will take you everywhere you want to go for the rest of your life.

PART I

Learn to Love Your Feet

1

An Inside Look at Your Feet

Approximately one and a half million years ago, *Homo erectus*— the first of our primate forebears to walk upright—appeared on Earth. That historic transition, which freed up two hands for such useful tasks as manipulating tools and (hundreds of thousands of years later) lighting fires and planting crops, also placed unprecedented demands on the spine, legs, and feet. If you entered the new millennium with sore feet or an aching back, you have those very distant ancestors—the ones who decided it was more convenient and more fun to stand up instead of crouching on all fours—to thank and to blame.

With two appendages bearing the weight nature originally assigned to four paws, it's not surprising that the foot has turned out to be one of the most vulnerable parts of the human body. The anatomy of the foot and ankle has evolved in ways that make it possible for us to engage in a variety of activities far more mechanically complicated than the clumping around and lunging of our prehistoric relatives. *Homo erectus* definitely never went skateboarding, performed a pirouette on point, landed a triple axel on the ice, played mixed doubles, or skipped rope double Dutch style.

The Renaissance artist and scientist Leonardo da Vinci rightly described the foot as both a "masterpiece of engineering and a work of art." This complex and delicate anatomical marvel consists of twenty-eight bones, thirty-five joints, fifty-six ligaments, and thirty-eight muscles—all needed to support the body's full weight. Feet are the final recipients of every pound of pressure imposed by every upright activity.

For its flexibility, the foot depends on the equally delicate ankle joint, with an Achilles tendon that must contract properly to provide the "pushoff" power for every step. That the foot and ankle work as well and as dependably as they do is a tribute to their strength and adaptability; that they sometimes break down, sending painful messages that they're in urgent need of attention, is the logical (though not inevitable) outcome of the heavy workload they bear.

With our first, shaky toddler steps, we begin a journey of at least 150,000 miles—the average distance a man or woman travels on foot in the course of a lifetime. But that's just a ballpark figure. A professional athlete can accumulate more than 300,000 miles. An amateur weekend tennis player—or even someone who walks an hour a day for exercise—is also adding tens of thousands of miles to the "average" lifetime burden.

THE LOAD WE BEAR

With every ordinary step, we place pressure on our feet equal to at least one and a half times our body weight, and the load increases sharply with even low-impact activities like brisk walking and ballroom dancing. High-impact exercise and sports, such as jogging, step aerobics, basketball, and tennis, can triple or quadruple the pressure.

Patients often ask me why walking imposes a burden that's actually heavier than their body weight. Climb onto a bathroom scale, and you'll see why. You don't step firmly onto the scale, do you? If you're like most people, you approach the dreaded measuring instrument in as gingerly a manner as possible, planting your feet while hanging onto a railing or vanity table, avoiding any excess motion while you transfer your entire weight to the scale itself. Without actually thinking about it, you're aware that any motion inflates your total weight tally. If you weigh 130 pounds standing motionless, you'd register 195 on the dial if you could walk back and forth across a large scale, and 390 if you could run on the same surface.

Here's the simple biomechanical equation determining the pressure we bear: Body weight plus intensity of impact equal the force that causes true wear and tear on the feet. That's one reason why adults tend to decrease their level of activity—sometimes without even realizing what they're doing—as they gain weight. With a twenty-pound weight gain, we put thirty extra pounds of pressure on our feet even when we're only walking at a slow pace. Running transforms that twenty pounds into sixty—and dozens of bones, joints, ligaments, and muscles must absorb the added impact. Bearing this mathematical formula in mind, it's easy to understand why so many overweight people become discouraged and give up on exercise.

A FOUNDATION OF BONES

If you consider the inner structure of the foot, it will be easier for you to understand the complexity of the mechanism that springs into action with each step. As a podiatrist, I'm awed by the elaborate design, and I find it something of a miracle that such a complicated assortment of bones and joints doesn't break down more often.

Your foot is divided into three basic sections: the forefoot, which includes the toes and the ball of the foot; the midfoot,

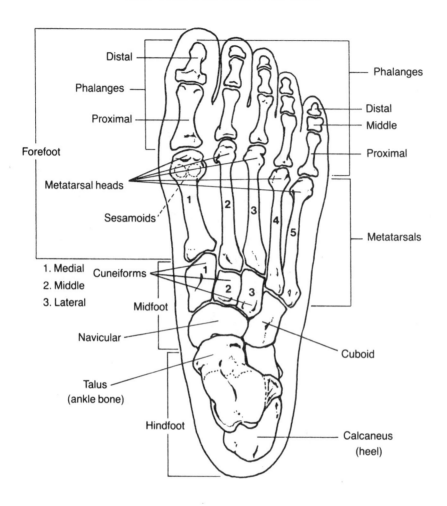

Figure 1. Bones of the foot (top view).

with an all-important arch that acts as a shock absorber for the entire body; and the hindfoot, with a heel and a triple joint linking your ankle to the arch in your midfoot. (See Figure 1.)

■ Fourteen small bones are joined together to make up your five toes (phalanges). The big toe (hallux) is composed of two bones, while each of the other toes is made up of three bones.

Interestingly, studies have shown that the average adult's little toe is smaller today than it was a century ago. We're not born that way (like every other body part, feet are bigger today as a result of improved nutrition), but many adults—especially women—alter the shape of their toes by squeezing the forefoot into too-narrow shoes. In Western countries before the twentieth century, only the tiny upper class—the one segment of society that didn't have to stand on its feet to make a living and could count on riding rather than walking—wore constricting shoes.

■ Also in the forefoot, two extremely tiny bones (sesamoids) lie buried at the base of the big toe. On X rays, the bones look like two eyeballs. The sesamoids are often ignored (some doctors even forget to mention them when they're talking about anatomy with patients), but they're extremely important: They act as pulleys for many muscles in the foot, and they also enable the big toe to move up and down. You've probably never heard of the sesamoid bones, but if you break one, you'll know it because you'll experience acute pain—and you probably won't be able to move your big toe.

■ The five long bones leading to each toe (metatarsals) complete the forefoot. Look at the top of your foot, and you can easily see the shape of these bones beneath the skin. The bottom side of the metatarsal area is the ball of your foot.

■ In the midfoot, five clumpy-looking, irregularly shaped bones (tarsals) make up your metatarsal arch (see Figure 2). This arch, linked to both the back and front of the foot by numerous muscles and the vital plantar fascia ligament—which connects the heel to the ball of your foot and is believed to be the strongest ligament in the body—provides the "spring" in your step. The higher the arch, the greater the spring.

Many people regard high-arched feet as "good" feet, but that judgment is based more on aesthetics—fashion photography has long exalted the high-arched woman—than on practical considerations. Like very low arches, extremely high arches have some drawbacks. For one thing, high arches place extra pressure on the heel, and that can cause stress fractures and pain in later life.

With age, the plantar fascia ligament loses some of its natural elasticity, causing most adults' arches—however high they were at birth—to flatten out to some degree. The shape of the tarsal bones, however, determines the original proportions of your arch.

■ The hindfoot encompasses your heel (calcaneus)—the largest bone in the foot—and your ankle bone (talus). The uniquely flexible ankle joint (subtalus) between the ankle and heel bones is a miracle of anatomy—a hinge that enables you to move your foot up and down and from side to side. Increasing the complexity—and the possibility for injury—is the fact that the ankle and heel bones also form joints with separate arch bones (see Figure 2). We're all triple-jointed at the back of our feet.

SOFT TISSUE: CONNECTING AND PADDING

The soft tissues in your foot include muscles, tendons, and ligaments too numerous to describe in detail. Ligaments are fibrous tissues that connect bones and help to stabilize joints; without them, your bones couldn't "cooperate" and enable you to walk.

I've already mentioned the importance of the plantar fascia ligament, a mighty band of tissue that links the back and the front bones of your foot. Even a minor strain in that ligament can cause considerable pain—not only in the soft tissue itself, but also in the bones that aren't getting their accustomed help.

Another critical soft tissue is the Achilles tendon, commonly called the heel cord, which you've probably heard of because it figures in so many injuries to prominent athletes.

Running along the back of the ankle, the heel cord is actually an extension of two major calf muscles, and it attaches your

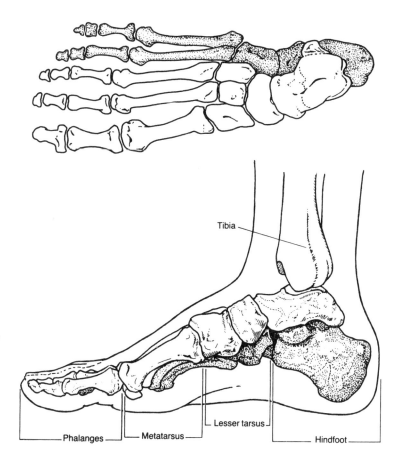

Figure 2. Functional units of the foot. The shaded areas provide support and the light areas are for shock absorption.

heel bone to the muscles (gastrocnemius and soleus) that make it possible for you to stand on tiptoes.

You probably know the story of Achilles from Greek mythology. His mother tried to render him invulnerable by dipping him as a baby into the waters of the River Styx, but she overlooked one spot—the heel she was clutching when she immersed the rest of her son. Due to his mom's oversight, Achilles was fatally wounded by a perfectly placed arrow during the Trojan War. I've always wondered whether that myth developed because ancient Greek runners, like runners today, wanted an explanation for the acute pain they experienced at the back of their ankles when they ran too far too fast.

Even though we're not conscious of "rising" on our toes when we walk normally, we're actually doing it imperceptibly with every step. Ordinary activities like climbing stairs, or athletic moves like jumping, give our Achilles tendons a more strenuous workout. Running is actually a series of small jumps, though that's not obvious to the naked eye.

Because the Achilles tendon is involved in every move we make, it's responsible for some of the most serious, difficult-to-treat foot and ankle injuries. For a professional athlete, a ruptured Achilles tendon can become a career-ending injury. Even for those who don't make exceptional athletic demands on their feet, a torn Achilles tendon may require months of rehabilitation.

THE FOOT IN MOTION

Walking—unlike, say, playing tennis—doesn't have to be taught. So it's not surprising that healthy adults don't give much thought to what actually happens when they put one foot in front of the other.

"Gait cycle" is the term podiatrists use to describe the action of the foot from the beginning to the end of each step, from heel strike to heel strike. Whenever something goes wrong with your foot, the gait cycle is inevitably disrupted.

When you're standing still, the back and the front of the foot bear equal weight, and your plantar fascia ligament, supporting the metatarsal arch, is in a relaxed position. As you begin your step, the weight shifts, and you strike the ground with the outer, back part of the heel.

Then the weight rolls forward toward the ball of the foot and big toe (these shifts all occur in a split second), while the plantar fascia ligament flattens out below the arch to help absorb the downward pressure. This necessary sagging of the ligament and metatarsal arch, as your weight shifts toward the forefoot, is called pronation.

Immediately after the midfoot makes solid contact with the ground, the weight shifts in the opposite direction (a process called supination). The foot lifts up, and you rise on your toes and the ball (here's where the Achilles tendon does its job). You push off, with your large thigh muscles helping to propel the body forward. Meanwhile, the plantar fascia ligament is contracting and curving slightly upward into the metatarsal arch. With this part of the gait cycle completed, your other foot is poised to begin its heel strike.

Ever wonder why the heels of your shoes wear down unevenly on one side or the other? If your foot rolls inward too much as your heel strikes the ground, you have a built-in mechanical glitch called overpronation. In underpronation, a less common flaw, the feet roll too far outward.

Overpronation is more likely to cause physical problems, because more pressure is shifted to the ball of the foot—which already carries 60 percent of the weight-bearing load in a person of normal gait. The muscles in your feet, calves, and even lower back must then work harder to compensate for the extra load imposed on the front of your foot.

YOUR PERSONAL GAIT

Think about how easy it is to recognize someone you know, even when you're not close enough to make out her features, by the way she walks. The gait of many celebrities and prominent historical figures is as famous as their faces: I can easily summon up images of Marilyn Monroe's swivel-hipped glide, Adolf Hitler's stiff-legged, herky-jerky motion, Queen Elizabeth II's short, neatly spaced, ladylike steps, Elvis Presley's gyrating progress across a stage. Everyone has a unique gait, and anything that feels comfortable is normal.

But many people wind up with what doctors call an antalgic gait, a pattern of walking that develops, often unconsciously, in an attempt to compensate for a physiological problem and avoid pain. Some antalgic gaits are the result of lower back or knee problems. Look at old films of President John F. Kennedy, who suffered from severe back pain for most of his adult life, and you'll notice his stiff, almost unnaturally upright walk—an obvious (to a physical therapist) attempt to minimize the pressure on his lower spine. I don't know whether Kennedy had time to worry about his feet, but his style of walking invariably causes foot pain in midlife. The weight can't shift easily back and forth between the heel and the forefoot as it does in the automatic, natural gait of a pain-free adult.

Other antalgic gaits work in reverse: They cause back and knee problems because you're trying to avoid a sore spot on your foot. Even something as small as a corn or blister—not to mention more significant bony deformities like bunions—can lead to back trouble because you're twisting yourself into a shape nature didn't intend as you try to keep the weight off that painful part of your foot.

When a new patient walks through my door, one of the first things I do is observe her as she walks across the room. Without asking a single question, I can almost always tell where the pain is.

After this inside look at your feet and your walking style, I hope you'll have a new appreciation of the intricacy of the mechanism that keeps you moving through life—and of the reasons why even a small podiatric problem can cause such intense pain. Some of us have inherited a foot structure that predisposes us to certain problems. My extremely flat feet, for example, made it likely that I would develop bunions at a relatively early age. But the way we walk—our gait—is a product not only of anatomy but also of life choices. A police officer who's on her feet most of the day inevitably develops a gait different from that of an executive who spends most of her time sitting at a desk. A woman who generally wears three-inch heels sways and minces because her shoes don't allow her to take long strides. Footwear, not just anatomy, determines the fate of our feet.

If your feet are chronically sore, chances are you're suffering from a combination of problems: those buried within the inherited structure of your foot, and those you've created for yourself through inattention and misuse. Both types of foot troubles are eminently solvable, but both worsen with age unless you start to pay more attention to your feet as you move into your thirties, forties, and beyond.

2

The Life Cycle of the Foot

Our feet, like the rest of our bodies, have a natural life cycle. Although hereditary bone deformities may cause trouble even for toddlers, the overwhelming majority of foot problems in adulthood are the result of our failure to understand and make allowances for the *normal* changes that affect our feet as we age. While many of my patients describe the onset of excruciating pain as "sudden," I usually find, in the course of taking a careful history, that they've ignored minor foot pain for years.

Lisa, a slender, physically active woman in her early forties—she takes regular dance classes and is the mother of a young son—first consulted me because, as she put it, she had developed acute pain in her feet "overnight." She admitted that she hadn't paid much attention to the mild soreness she'd been experiencing for years during her customary long walks. When I looked at the soles of her feet, I saw a purplish discoloration that Lisa hadn't even noticed. Her feet were actually being bruised—and bruised deeply and painfully—by their constant contact with the unyielding cement sidewalks of New York City.

I told Lisa something she hadn't known: By the forties,

everyone has lost some of the fatty cushion that protects the ball of the foot. By the 75,000-mile mark—which fitness-conscious people like Lisa reach well before those who lead more sedentary lives—as much as half of the fatty tissue has been lost. And Lisa's feet were taking an extra pounding because she frequently walked in ballerina flats, which have less padding on the bottom than nearly all other women's shoes.

For pain caused by this predictable kind of age-related change, the solution is laughably simple: Buy shoes with more cushioning and add a padded insole or orthotic for sports and exercise. "It really didn't occur to me that this level of pain could be caused by something so simple," Lisa told me. "You look in the mirror and see a gray hair and you know it's the result of getting older. But you don't think of feet as having an age. They're just—well, they're just your feet."

If you want to walk fluidly and comfortably throughout your life—and who doesn't?—you must learn to understand, respect, and accommodate your health and fitness habits to the foot's "biological clock."

BIRTH TO THIRTY: THE FOOTLOOSE YEARS

When they hold a newborn baby in their arms, one of the first things most parents do is count the number of fingers and toes. Something about those perfect little hands and feet is especially endearing: Long after teenagers are gallumphing around in their oversize athletic shoes, most mothers have the tiny booties tucked away somewhere in a drawer.

And most children's feet are indeed perfect, a perfect work in progress. On an X ray, a child's foot appears to have many more bones than an adult's. That's because the bones continue growing not only in infancy, childhood, and the early teen years but also in late adolescence. The skeletal structure of the foot is not fully knitted together until we're nearly twenty. The apparent gaps on a child's X ray are occupied by cartilage that will be completely replaced by solid bone only when the foot is fully formed.

Fortunately, most of the problems parents worry about are perfectly normal stages in the development of a baby's and child's foot. (For the exceptions, see Chapter 4, "Your Children's Feet.") Many parents consult me because they're convinced that their toddlers have "flat" feet. In fact, all toddlers' feet look flat because of the thick fatty pad that obscures the arch. (This "baby fat" is part of what makes those little feet look so adorable.)

The fat cushioning begins to disappear when a child learns to walk, and a visible arch normally appears around the time of a child's fourth birthday. If she really does turn out to have abnormally flat feet, there's nothing lost by waiting to begin treatment until age four—something doctors didn't know when I was growing up.

It's also perfectly normal for children to be somewhat bow-legged until age two, knock-kneed between ages two and four, and slightly bowed again from four to six. The changing stance of young children is usually a natural and healthy accommodation to growth and weight shifts.

Of course, a parent should consult a podiatrist if she's worried about her child's gait. Precisely because bowed legs and knock-knees are so common and generally so harmless, even an excellent pediatrician may miss signs of an uncommon knee or foot problem that a podiatrist would recognize. If there's nothing wrong with the child—and that's usually the case—a visit to a podiatrist will set the parent's mind at rest.

I'll never forget the day when two anxious mothers had scheduled appointments for their seven-year-old daughters on the same morning. One of the girls had bowed legs, and the other had knock-knees. When I walked into the waiting room to call in the first mother-daughter pair, the two girls were standing next to each other and giggling unrestrainedly. They had just discovered that they could spell out OX with their legs by standing side by side. There wasn't anything wrong with either girl. In most instances, these minor knee deviations (in either direction) correct themselves, without treatment, by age eight.

Young Adults

Throughout childhood and adolescence, most healthy children enjoy every kind of activity on pain-free feet. Because foot pain in the young is the exception rather than the rule, any sustained discomfort merits a visit to the doctor to rule out the possibility of an undetected injury.

Teenagers, in particular, are apt to minimize pain and ignore the possibility of injury because they don't want to interrupt their usual routine. At sixteen, a friend of mine walked around for a month on an agonizingly sore toe, without telling her parents, because she was scheduled to take her driver's license test and was afraid she'd have to put it off if a doctor got a look at her foot. When she owned up to the pain (the day after receiving her license), it turned out that she'd broken her toe during a volleyball game. Because the break had started to heal in the wrong position, the toe had to be rebroken and set in a hard cast—and my friend was on crutches for a month.

The Twenties

For most people, the twenties basically mean more of the same for feet. If you've had healthy feet as a child and a teenager, that's not likely to change in your twenties.

When I treat people in their twenties, they're generally suffering from an exercise-related injury or minor infections (either viral warts or funguses) picked up in nail parlors or the locker room of a health club. If they're in good general health, their feet are healthy too. Around thirty, that begins to change. The rest of the body may be in great shape, but feet begin to show the wear and tear of their responsibility as our ultimate weight-bearers.

THE THIRTIES: FROM FOOTLOOSE TO FOOTSORE

In a scary science fiction movie called *Logan's Run*, everyone in an isolated domed city is vaporized at age thirty-two. Those who don't want to enter the next world at such a young age are forced to run for their lives in order to escape the confines of their sealed universe. The screenwriter picked exactly the right cutoff age, because if the city's inhabitants had been scheduled for vaporization at forty, few of them would have been quick enough on their feet to get away.

Four out of five of my patients are over thirty. While there are always individual exceptions, the basic difference between thirty-five-year-old and twenty-five-year-old feet is in the elasticity of the ligaments, muscles, and tendons. Feet become more vulnerable to all types of injury (especially during exercise) because these soft tissues tighten up and sometimes go into spasm instead of working smoothly to allow free movement.

I've worked with a number of professional athletes, and all of them report that it takes longer to "get loose" in their thirties than it did in their twenties. An athlete over thirty also requires more rest for the muscles to rebound after strenuous effort. If you're a baseball fan, you know that managers often rest their veteran players—the "senior citizens" in their early thirties—when the team plays a day game after a night game.

If pro athletes need more R & R in their thirties, that's even more true of the average thirtysomething man or woman. This is the decade when many people decide it's time to "get back in shape"—the shape they remember from college or even high school, before they sat behind a desk for years or went through pregnancy and childbirth. If they're like Roger, a thirty-year-old stockbroker who came limping into my office one morning last spring, they've tried to jump back immediately into the routine they followed when they were ten years younger and twenty pounds lighter. (Weight gain is a factor in many foot troubles in the thirties.)

Roger, who played baseball in both high school and college, decided it was time to take off twenty pounds and regain his old athletic form. He started playing ball in Central Park without doing warm-ups and immediately developed intense shooting pains, between the kneecap and ankle, known as shin splints. These pains are caused by a pulling away from the bone of the anterior tibial muscles in front of the leg (which enable you to lift up your toes). These are called antigravity muscles, because (unlike the back muscles in your calf) they aren't developed automatically by walking.

"I never used to warm up," Roger grumbled when I recommended a series of careful stretching exercises before he returned to a baseball diamond. "Used to," I told him, was the operative phrase. Thirty obviously isn't ancient, but it's not twenty.

Once you understand and accept the need for extra stretching and conditioning in the thirties, you shouldn't have any trouble with the physical activities enjoyed by people in their teens and twenties. In fact, I urge all of my sedentary patients over thirty to increase their activity level as soon as possible. If you haven't been continuously active as a young adult, it's better to begin an exercise program sooner rather than later. Start a fitness program in your early thirties, and you may never develop the painful foot problems that plague people who wait until they're nearing their fiftieth birthday to "get back in shape."

Some women also begin to develop visible bunions in their

thirties. The bunions don't necessarily hurt, though many women dislike the appearance of their feet and are beginning to have trouble finding comfortable shoes. In the thirties, a change of footwear—away from pointed-toed high heels—may be all that's needed to slow the development of the bunion and avoid surgery in later years. Women who do need bunion surgery in their thirties are the exception rather than the rule. In most such cases, the woman inherited a foot structure that produced the beginnings of bunions in adolescence.

Early Warnings of Other Health Problems

Finally—and I can't stress this enough—the foot in the thirties also serves as an early-warning system for age-related, systemic diseases that may not manifest themselves in the rest of the body until the forties, fifties, or even sixties. Because the feet are literally our extremities—farthest from the heart—they are the first body parts to display signs of impaired circulation.

When a patient complains about chronically cold feet, for instance, she almost always turns out to be a smoker. For that reason, patients can't lie to me about their smoking habit: I can make an educated guess about the number of cigarettes they smoke each day not only from their foot temperature but from the color of the skin (grayish-white instead of a healthy pink).

As is well known, smoking impairs blood circulation, both by causing the blood vessels to constrict and by clogging them with tar and nicotine residue. Long before the cumulative impact of smoking places you at higher risk for stroke and heart attack, your cold feet may be warning you that the process of circulatory impairment has already begun. That such signs of future trouble appear in the thirties is a blessing rather than a curse: There is still plenty of time to halt—and in many instances reverse—the damage inflicted by poor health habits.

In the late thirties, many people also develop the first signs of arthritis. These arthritic changes may complicate other conditions, like bunions, that haven't caused any pain in the past. Since age-related osteoarthritis (the most common form of the disease) is basically an inflammation of the cartilage and lining of the joints, the foot—with its thirty-five extremely small joints—often develops symptoms before the rest of the body. Systemic rheumatoid arthritis, a far more serious and much less common form of the disease, may also declare itself for the first time in the thirties.

THE FORTIES: AGING BABY BOOMERS

In the forties, the shock absorbers in the foot begin to go. General pain in the heel, arch, and ball of the foot—even in the absence of a specific injury—is the most common complaint of my patients between forty and fifty. Like Lisa, who didn't realize that she'd lost much of the fatty padding beneath her foot, these patients feel pain in their feet whenever they walk.

As I've already indicated, ligaments, muscles, and other soft tissues tighten up somewhat in the thirties. In the forties, the tissues also slacken and loosen. This sounds contradictory, but it really isn't. Your soft tissues are losing some of their overall elasticity: Not only do they have more of a tendency to go into spasm when they contract, but they don't retain as much firmness during the relaxation part of the gait cycle.

I prefer to use words like "relax" and "slacken" because they sound so much more appealing than "sag." In truth, though, our feet—like the rest of our bodies—do start to sag and spread out in the forties. That's why we call arches "fallen."

It's perfectly normal for feet to spread out at this age, and it's a rare person who doesn't need a larger shoe at fifty than at forty. By fifty, most of us should be wearing shoes a full size larger than we did at twenty. While men generally buy bigger shoes without giving the decision a second thought, women frequently cling to their teen shoe size. That's a mistake. Clothing manufacturers have accommodated to the youthful self-image of aging boomer women by "downsizing" clothes (today's size 8 was our mother's size 10 or 12), but shoe manufacturers haven't changed their sizing. Today's 7B was yesterday's 7B; only the size of our feet has changed if the shoe doesn't fit. (Of course, you may manage to find a shoe brand that tends to "run large.")

✗ Comfortable shoes and regular stretching and strengthening exercises for the heel cord and lower leg muscles are the key to foot fitness in the forties.

THE FIFTIES: DEADLINE DECADE

In their fifties, my patients are old enough to begin thinking seriously about what they need to do to remain physically fit and maintain their wide range of activities for the rest of their

Your Genetic and Cultural Inheritance

By your forties and fifties, your feet are beginning to show the results not only of the way you've lived but also of your genetic heritage. For the most part, my African-American patients have wider, flatter feet than whites (especially whites of northern European descent). This means that blacks are more likely to have fallen arches and to need orthotics at an earlier age than people of other ethnic and racial groups. On the other hand, African-American women are much less likely to develop osteoporosis than whites: At an age when many white women begin to experience stress fractures in their heels, I rarely see a problem among my black patients.

My Latina patients fall somewhere between blacks and whites on the bone density scale. Many of them have severe bunions, but I suspect this has more to do with the admiration for high-heeled women in Latin culture than it does with hereditary bone structure. "I wasn't allowed to wear high heels until my fifteenth birthday party, which is like your sweet sixteen," explained a beautiful forty-eight-year-old Cuban American with two of the worst bunions I've ever seen. "I picked out four-inch heels for my first grown-up party, and I've worn at least three-inch heels my whole life. Now you're telling me I have to change my whole idea of what's pretty if I'm ever going to walk without pain again. Well, I guess that's better than the wheelchair."

I suspect that these ethnic differences will become less pronounced if the number of racial and ethnic intermarriages continues to increase throughout our country. But you should be aware that both your genetic and cultural heritage are likely to play a role in the foot problems you develop in midlife.

lives. The oldest baby boomers, born in 1946, will turn fifty-five next year, and they have completely different attitudes about fitness and aging than the fifty-five-year-old patients I treated when I opened my practice in 1980.

Loss of fatty padding under the ball of the foot, which first manifests itself in the forties, continues in the fifties. For reasons that aren't fully understood, the tissue deterioration seems to accelerate after the the 75,000-mile mark—an important point for fitness and exercise enthusiasts to remember. I believe that everyone over fifty should use a special orthotic insole while engaging in any form of weight-bearing exercise—any movement that creates an impact between your foot and the ground. Walking, running, and step aerobics are examples of weight-bearing activities. Non-weight-bearing exercise, such as swimming, is often recommended for people with joint problems in their knees, ankles, and feet. I've found, though, that most people in their fifties and sixties can enjoy both types of exercise if they wear protective shoes and don't overdo it.

Not only does the internal fatty padding thin out, the outer layer of skin also thins and dries out in the fifties. This can cause painful cracks and heel fissures, which serve as portals for all types of viral and bacterial infections, so it's important to pamper the skin with moisturizing creams. Women are already accustomed to moisturizing their skin, and most are aware that menopause-associated loss of estrogen leads to drier skin on every area of the body. But I sometimes have trouble convincing my male patients—even when they walk in with bleeding fissures in their heels—that their skin also needs extra attention. "Male menopause" isn't marked by an obvious event like the end of menstruation, but age-related hormonal changes also affect men's skin and fatty tissues. Interestingly, men take to foot pampering with great enthusiasm after I convince them to try the unscented medicated creams that I mix in my office. Not only do the fissures heal, but several men have confessed in embarrassed tones that they like the way their feet *look* under the new regime.

For women in the years just before, during, and immediately after menopause, tiny hairline fractures in the bones of the heels and toes (painful but sometimes invisible on conventional X rays) may be the first sign of low bone density, which can lead to full-blown osteoporosis in the seventies and eighties. Only last year, a special low-dose X ray that measures bone density in feet became available for use in doctors' offices. I recommend this inexpensive ($50–$100) evaluation, known as "peripheral" testing, to every female patient over fifty. If the test reveals low bone density, I urge the woman to consult her gynecologist about hormone replacement therapy, dietary changes, and exercises designed to preserve bone. This offers yet another example of the ways feet can provide an early indicator of changes in the rest of the body.

FITNESS AFTER FIFTY

When I began practicing twenty years ago, I saw relatively few patients in their fifties (unless they were retired pro athletes) with recurring foot and ankle problems attributable to old sports injuries. That's no longer the case: The baby boomers now entering their fifties are the first generation to have exercised—and sometimes overexercised—throughout their adult lives. The late 1970s and early 1980s were the Age of the Runner, and many of my patients pulled tendons and tore ligaments by "going for the burn" and "playing through the pain." Although they recovered from these injuries with little difficulty, as people generally do in their twenties and thirties, they've been left with a heightened vulnerability to reinjury in the same old spot.

One of the challenges for fitness-conscious men and women in their fifties is maintaining a satisfying exercise routine while making realistic accommodations to the age of their joints and the aftereffects of past injuries. I try to help patients custom-design an exercise program that meets their psychological and emotional needs while respecting their physical limitations. Should you jog five miles a day on a badly arthritic ankle and fallen arches? No. Can you achieve the same fitness results through a combination of shorter runs and other exercises? Absolutely.

Of course, some men and women in their fifties have precisely the opposite problem: They've decided—often after being told by a doctor that they need to lower their blood pressure and cholesterol level—that it's time to abandon the sedentary habits of a lifetime. For those just beginning to exercise at this age, it's particularly important to find the right cushioned footwear and to learn how to stretch the muscles to avoid soft-tissue injuries—even before such seemingly harmless activities as brisk walking.

SIXTY-PLUS

A sixty-year-old woman today can expect to live to age eighty-two, a man to age seventy-nine. When I see patients in this age group, I'm often reminded of what the feminist activist and writer Gloria Steinem said on her fortieth birthday when someone complimented her on her youthful appearance. "This is what forty looks like," Steinem replied.

In their sixties, my patients seem to live basically the same lives they did in their fifties, with a little more leisure thrown into the mix. Unless they have serious systemic health problems—and most don't—they're usually able to carry on with the same fitness routines they established in the previous decade.

Many Americans make more demands on their feet in the sixties than they did when they were younger. A study last year by the American Association of Retired Professionals found that the proportion of men who engaged in daily exercise, such as brisk walking or cycling, was 40 percent higher in the sixty-to-seventy-four age group than for those between forty-five and sixty. For women, the proportion of exercisers jumped by 25 percent over sixty. Looking at those figures, it's obvious that pain-free feet are a vital component of the increasingly active lifestyles of people in this age group.

THE SURGICAL DECADE

The incidence of foot surgery on women peaks in the sixties. Many have lived with painful bunions or hammertoes since their thirties, and they're aware that today's surgical techniques have greatly shortened recovery time. Also, I find that people in their sixties are generally more eager than thirty-year-olds to deal aggressively with a medical condition that can be corrected. "I don't have time for this," said a sixty-one-year-old woman whose bunion had long prevented her from running and was now interfering with ordinary walking. "Every day I can't move in exactly the way I want to is a day I can't get back."

Although foot surgery has been performed with great success on people in their seventies and even late eighties, I urge patients in their sixties to act sooner rather than later if foot pain is restricting their everyday activities. If an operation is the only way to rid yourself of pain, it makes no sense to wait. As is well known, the body takes longer to heal after injury or surgery with every passing year.

Because people over sixty are more likely to suffer from impaired blood circulation, they're also more likely to need regular podiatric care. Fifteen percent of the over-sixty-five population has diabetes, which impairs blood flow and leaves the lower extremities extremely vulnerable to infection. Other circulation-impairing conditions with a higher incidence in this age group include lupus and rheumatoid arthritis. I can't stress enough that if you've been diagnosed with any disease that compromises blood circulation, you should take care of even the most routine foot problems—calluses, corns, cracked heels—in a sterile medical setting. You can't afford to expose yourself to bacterial contamination that lurks in nail parlors with inadequate sanitary precautions.

Of course, ordinary degenerative arthritis is the chief complaint of people in their sixties, seventies, and beyond. As a podiatrist, my goal is the same as that of my patients: to keep them on their feet at every age. For physically active people in their sixties and seventies, my recommendations are virtually the same as they were in the thirties and forties: stretching exercises, padded shoes, orthotic insoles for weight-bearing activities. The only difference is that you need to spend more time "getting loose," something people accept more readily in their sixties than they did in their thirties.

During the past decade, every medical study has found a close link between exercise and health (mental and physical) in older Americans. Are these people healthier because they exercise, or do they exercise more because they're already healthy? "Both" is my answer. While my older patients do cut back on exercise when they're sick, I'm amazed at the important role that ordinary walking plays in recovery from even the most serious heart and cancer surgeries.

"I'm back on my feet" is an important statement of emotional as well as physical well-being. As a doctor, I love hearing these words—and I expect to hear them—from people of every age.

3

Double Standard:
The Love-Hate Relationship
Between Women and Their Feet

"I hate my feet." It's an opening line I hear from many women who are consulting a podiatrist for the first time. Although these women may have lived with foot pain for years, they're usually talking about the way their feet look rather than the way they feel. Some are so embarrassed about visible bunions and discolored nails that they've always taken great pains to avoid letting anyone—including a lover—get a close look at their feet and toes. You'd think nothing else could embarrass a woman who's lying on a gynecologist's examining table with her feet in stirrups, but many patients have told me how mortified they were when they realized that they were wearing transparent knee-highs, giving the doctor a clear view (in the unlikely event that he should wish to take a close look) of their discolored toenails, corns, and bunions.

But this concern with appearance isn't a matter of pure vanity. There's frequently a direct connection between the way feet look and smell and the way they feel (something I often have to explain to men). Female concern about the appearance of feet is a reflection of the greater prevalence of visually unappealing, and sometimes medically serious, joint and toe problems in women. Sore feet are not equal opportunity tormenters.

Walk into any podiatric surgeon's waiting room, and you'll see that the majority of patients are women. In my own practice, women outnumber men four to one. Across the nation, women account for nearly nine out of ten surgeries performed to correct bony deformities like bunions and hammertoes. A study by the American Orthopaedic Foot and Ankle Society (AOFAS), a professional organization of M.D. orthopedists specializing in foot disorders, has estimated that foot and ankle surgery on women costs $3.5 billion each year and is responsible for fifteen million lost work days annually.

My male patients tend to be middle-aged "weekend warriors" who've pulled up lame after trying to transform themselves instantly from couch potatoes into the athletes they used to be (or imagined themselves to be). They've done something *special* to injure their feet. My women patients, by contrast, are usually suffering from chronic pain even during everyday activities—pain they've mistakenly come to regard as "normal."

What accounts for the enormous gender gap in podiatric problems? Shoes, as I've already indicated, are an important contributing factor, but they're not the whole explanation. I'm living proof, with bunions that began developing when I was a little girl in orthopedic oxfords, that sensible shoes can't prevent structural and biomechanical foot trouble in anyone whose heredity predisposes her (or him) to bony deformities. Male or female, if one of your parents had a bunion in adolescence or early adulthood, you're more likely to develop one too. And if both of your parents had early bunions, you're a sitting (excuse me, walking) duck for the same problem. Some people can wear spike heels for a lifetime without ever developing a blister, much less a bunion, while others—those with the hereditary predisposition—would develop unsightly, painful bumps even if they strolled barefoot on sandy beaches from birth to old age.

FEET AND HORMONES

Women not only have a higher incidence of bony deformities but also are especially vulnerable to tendon and ligament injuries. Throughout the body, women's ligaments are more flexible than men's—an elasticity that serves us well during pregnancy and childbirth but can cause foot and knee trouble at any age. The immense flood of estrogen during pregnancy (and, to a lesser degree, the regular hormonal shifts of the menstrual cycle) encourages the loosening of ligaments still further. During the 1990s, as more women have begun to participate in high-impact sports, it has also become apparent that even the most physically fit young women are more prone to knee and ankle injuries than their equally athletic male counterparts. Flexible ligaments give us a wider range of motion than men in many of our joints, but they also destabilize our knees and ankles.

Rapid weight gain also encourages slack ligaments. The permanent stretch marks on the abdomens of many mothers offer visible evidence of the fact that ligaments don't always snap firmly back into place even after a woman has regained her prepregnancy weight. Ligaments in the feet don't always snap back either, but most women, if they wear shoes with proper support during pregnancy, won't have any special problems afterward.

What does affect feet over the long run is yo-yo dieting, in which a woman loses, regains, loses, and regains significant amounts of weight dozens of times in the course of a lifetime. What amount of weight is significant for feet? Ten pounds, if you gain and lose it often enough, can permanently overstretch ligaments. Pregnancy, for most American women today, is a twice-in-a-lifetime event—but there's no limit to the number of diets we can try.

Loss of bone mass after menopause, as I've noted, also places women over fifty at greater risk for stress fractures of the foot. And, of course, women of every age have smaller bones than men. The "well-turned ankle," as our grandfathers used to call it, is a slender ankle, and slim ankles are inherently more prone to sprains and breaks than the thicker, serviceable-looking joints connecting men's feet to their calves. I often treat women who've badly hurt an ankle while simply stepping off a curb the wrong way (even while wearing flat walking shoes).

FEMININE OVERLOAD

There's another frequently overlooked factor in the pounding endured by women's feet: We're the everyday "beasts of burden" of our species. Waiting at a bus stop around 5:30, I observe a young woman wearing high heels and an elegant business suit and struggling with everything she's carrying as she gets off the bus. She has a huge purse slung over her left shoulder (I read somewhere that the contents of the average woman's bag weigh more than five pounds), a briefcase in her left hand, and two shopping bags from grocery and department stores in her right hand. The men getting off the bus are carrying briefcases. Period. On the same corner is another woman with an equally weighty load—except she's also balancing a baby and a stroller she intends to lug onto the bus. As far as feet are concerned, there's no difference between body weight and the weight of whatever we're carrying: It all translates into pressure on the ball of the foot. On any given day, the extra "toting" weight doesn't matter much; over a lifetime, it adds up to more wear and tear on women's feet.

CINDERELLA'S SHOES

How much does women's long love affair with the wrong shoes contribute to foot problems? Shoes emphatically do not *cause* major deformities like bunions, but they can and do aggravate structural problems—and speed up the degenerative process that, in the most painful cases, leaves surgery as the only option.

Furthermore, shoes greatly exacerbate the biomechanical component of a painful gait. What podiatrists mean by biomechanics is the way your weight shifts on your feet as you walk. Remember pronation? If your foot is overpronated, your weight doesn't shift evenly from your heel to the ball of your foot. Your big toe—and the first metatarsal joint where bunions emerge—must bear too much pressure.

The wrong shoes (see Chapter 22, "Shoe Savvy," for advice on finding the right ones) intensify biomechanical imbalances in several ways. Here's how the process works. A two-inch heel imposes two and a half times more pressure on the ball of your foot than a three-quarter-inch heel. The extra pressure exceeds the elevation because the added height changes the angle of your foot, placing more weight on a smaller surface. Put on four-inch spikes or platform heels, and you're putting five times as much pressure on the forefoot. The extreme example of forefoot stress is a ballerina on pointe: The entire weight of the body (multiplied many times by the difficult high-impact moves that make classical ballet so beautiful) descends not on the ball of the foot but on the toes themselves. Badly deformed feet are a price female dancers inevitably—and gladly—pay for the love of their calling, but I never watch the vision of grace and loveliness on stage without thinking of the twisted bones and infected blisters I've treated in my examining room.

Most women, of course, aren't dancers, and most of us won't develop any extra foot problems as a result of occasionally wearing spike heels in the evening. But even relatively conservative two-inch heels (which millions of women, including me, wear to work) have a cumulative impact on anyone with a hereditary tendency toward painful foot problems. I always shift to lower-heeled shoes when I'm performing surgery, but many working women—think of the huge number on their feet all day in retail sales establishments—lack that option.

Do women know that high heels aren't good for their feet? Of course they do—and growing numbers of younger women are acting on that awareness. Studies have shown that women under thirty are most likely to wear athletic shoes and least likely to wear high heels to work. (These findings could be misleading, though, because young women who haven't completed their education are more likely to work at nonprofessional jobs in which casual clothes are accepted.) Ironically, women in their forties and fifties—the very age at which joint deformities are likely to become painful—are most likely to spend the work day in high heels.

What many women don't know, though, is they may be inflicting pain on themselves—and nurturing bunions and hammertoes—by wearing shoes, regardless of heel height, that are too narrow in front. A nationwide survey by AOFAS found that 88 percent of women squeeze their feet into shoes that are, on an average, a half inch too narrow. Most fashionable shoes measure only about three inches across at their widest point, while most women's feet measure between three and a half and four inches.

These too-narrow shoes must be "broken in"—and the only way we break in shoes is by rubbing our bones and soft tissue against the leather until it finally gives us relief. Or until we shove them into the back of the closet. Men buy shoes to fit their feet, while we Cinderellas try to make our feet fit our shoes; a shoe, like a bra, becomes an instrument to rearrange our natural assets into a more fashionable and (we often think) sexier shape. In this respect, the wrong shoes not only aggravate structural and biomechanical problems but also encourage the love-hate relationship between women and their feet.

To sum up, the female bone structure, hormonal system, and high-fashion shoes set women up for many more foot and ankle problems than the majority of men will ever experience.

I want my women patients to accept their feet—to realize that working with what nature has given them, instead of trying to squeeze into the glass slipper, is the way to improve both the appearance and the health of this indispensable part of the body.

PART II

Common and Uncommon Complaints

4

Athlete's Foot

WHAT GOES WRONG?

Athlete's foot is the most common fungal infection in both adults and children. Its clinical name, *tinea pedis*, literally means "grubs, larva, or worms" in the skin. You definitely don't need to be an athlete to contract a fungus. Moist locker rooms and nonbreathing athletic shoes encourage the growth of these organisms, and unsanitary nail parlors are also a perfect breeding ground for funguses.

It's a rare adult who hasn't had a case of athlete's foot at some point in life. Pregnant women, people over sixty-five, and those with systemic immune disorders are especially vulnerable. Any condition that compromises the ability of your immune system to resist disease renders you more vulnerable to garden-variety funguses like *candida albicans*, one of the most common organisms responsible for athlete's foot.

If you come into a podiatrist's office complaining of an itching foot, she'll probably take a scraping of your skin and put it through a laboratory culture test to determine exactly which organism is responsible. (One reason for these cultures, also taken on fungus nails, is to determine whether a bacterial and/or a fungal infection is present. Also, the symptoms of athlete's foot may resemble those caused by warts, various skin allergies, and psoriasis, which require different treatments and medication.)

SYMPTOMS

- The area is covered with scaly, whitish patches. These may appear between your toes, on your heels, or anywhere on the soles of your feet.
- Intense itching is the most common sign of a more advanced case of athlete's foot. In general, the more you itch, the deeper the infection. Many early cases of athlete's foot don't itch at all.
- The skin may crack, with accompanying redness and an unpleasant odor.
- In severe cases that haven't been treated, the area becomes infected and oozes a white or yellow discharge. Needless to say, this hurts. If this happens, go see your doctor immediately.
- Sometimes, you may develop similar symptoms on your hand as a result of touching your foot. (This also happens with warts.)

UNMENTIONABLES: SWEAT AND SMELLS

Sometimes, people make the mistake of confusing athlete's foot with ordinary sweat that gives off a pungent odor. Sweat is, of course, your body's way of maintaining its even temperature regardless of what the temperature is outside. Yet many people are extremely, and unnecessarily, embarrassed about the way their feet smell. Patients frequently apologize to me, convinced that their foot odor is overpowering, while I'm examining them. I'm able to tell most of them that there's nothing unusual or particularly offensive about the odor of their feet. Believe me, I'd know!

A minority of people do suffer from truly excessive sweat production. *Bromhidrosis* is the technical medical term used to describe secretion of excessive and smelly sweat. The word is a compound of the Greek *bromos* ("stench") and *hidros* ("sweat"). This is not really a medical problem, though people often consult a podiatrist about it.

Only when the sweat is so excessive that it leads to the formation of blisters and encourages infection do we treat this condition medically. Then the condition is called *dyshidrosis*. In some cases, dyshidrosis is a sign of nerve damage, either as a result of trauma or a systemic disease affecting the nervous system. Normally (however sweaty your feet feel), the amount of sweat is so small that it can't even be measured. Unlucky people with dyshidrosis may produce as much as a pint of sweat a week. In these cases, a podiatrist may prescribe a drug that blocks the impulses in your nervous system that are producing excess perspiration. There is also a new antiperspirant medication called Botox that is injected directly into the soles of the feet.

In most cases, though, commonsense self-care is your best remedy. Change your shoes and socks frequently. Don't wear shoes with synthetic material that traps the sweat inside. Sometimes people use underarm deodorants and antiperspirants on their feet. There's nothing wrong with this if sweat is your only problem, but these products can be harmful if you have blisters or other foot infections. Frequent washing and drying, and powdering with ordinary cornstarch after the feet are thoroughly dry, is probably your best bet.

You should definitely consult a podiatrist if your excessive sweat production is accompanied by some of the symptoms I've listed for athlete's foot. If what you need is antibacterial cream, you shouldn't be putting deodorant on your feet. Also, you should never use the same deodorant stick on your feet and your underarms because you might be transporting a foot infection to your armpits. Yes, it's a nasty thought—and you don't want it to happen to you.

FROM MY FILES

Most patients come in for treatment of athlete's foot when over-the-counter creams haven't worked. Unlike nail fungus, athlete's foot frequently does respond to nonprescription medications *if they're used as directed.* You must use creams rather than powders. Most of the brand-name creams are highly effective: Desenex, Halog, and Micatin are among the most common brands on drugstore shelves. The instructions on nearly all of these products recommend use for thirty days, but many people make the mistake of stopping the medication in a week or two, when the visible symptoms disappear. The same rule applies as with oral antibiotics: Take it all, even if you feel better midway through the treatment.

When self-care doesn't work, the next step is to see a doctor for specific tests to determine exactly what's causing your problem. The treatment is quite straightforward and standard. In most instances, I recommend a stronger prescription cream that must also be used for a month. If the laboratory culture shows that there's also a bacterial infection, an oral antibiotic may be needed.

Untreated fungus can lead to deep fissures in the skin, and the inflamed fissures serve as ports of entry for bacteria that can spread throughout your system.

Pam, an aerobics enthusiast in her early thirties, ignored her itching and the increasingly inflamed cracks in her heels until she saw a puslike fluid around the fissures. In fact, the fluid *was* pus, and Pam wound up in the hospital, receiving antibiotics through an IV to combat a serious case of bacterial cellulitis. This is obviously a rare example, but it demonstrates the importance of treating itchy athlete's foot before it encourages other types of opportunistic infections. I can't emphasize enough that if there's any redness, swelling, or discharge associated with what you think is a case of ordinary athlete's foot, you should see your doctor immediately.

PREVENTION AND SELF-CARE

■ Never—I mean *never*—walk around barefoot in a locker room or any other damp environment in which you don't know whose germs you're sharing. If you share a bathroom with someone who already has athlete's foot, keep those shower clogs handy.

■ Don't wear the same socks home from the gym that you wore to work out. Always keep a fresh, clean pair of socks in your gym bag or locker. Damp socks are a perfect medium for carrying fungal organisms from your health club to your home. And stick to white socks, because dyes encourage fungal growth.

■ Bring your own instruments to nail parlors and use an antifungal agent, like Betadine solution, in basins where you soak your feet. Athlete's foot can be contracted as easily in a nail parlor as in a locker room.

■ Don't wear athletic shoes all day. Unlike leather, the synthetic materials used in most athletic shoes don't allow your feet to "breathe." Spend part of your day in shoes made of natural materials and expose your feet to sunlight and air as much as possible.

Other people may make fun of you for your hgyienic precautions. Do you really care? Which would you rather do—put on rubber clogs every time you walk into a locker room or suffer from a maddening itch for weeks?

■ I recommend two home remedies for extremely sweaty feet. Sprinkle the insides of your shoes liberally with talcum powder or cornstarch, which absorb sweat. Before you go out, have a very cold five-minute footbath, followed by a very hot soak. Then fix yourself a third footbath of ice cubes and lemon juice. Finally, rub your feet with alcohol, dry them, and slip them into your powdered shoes. This procedure really works: It reduces perspiration by constricting the blood flow. In hot weather, I recommend that you follow this routine every day. You'll find that this does more to make your feet feel cool and dry than any commercial deodorant.

■ A second home remedy involves a mixture of a half cup of kosher salt (which has larger crystals than ordinary table salt) per quart of water. Soak your feet in the lukewarm solution for five minutes. And don't forget to powder your shoes with corn-starch or talcum powder.

5

Bunions

WHAT GOES WRONG?

"Bunions!" exclaimed thirty-seven-year-old Heather in a disgusted voice. "Even the word is ugly. Couldn't you call it something else?" Alas, the word was intended to encompass both pain and ugliness. The English word is derived from the French and Italian (*bugnone, bugno*), meaning "boil" or "lump." It appears in the kind of medieval literature describing the tortures of the damned, and no one who has ever suffered from a badly inflamed bunion would disagree.

The classic bunion is a bony protrusion on the outside of the big toe, accompanied in adults by degenerative arthritic changes in the bone underneath. Bunionettes are petite cousins on the outside of the little toe. Both bunions and bunionettes normally come in pairs, even though the development in one foot is generally more advanced than in the other.

There are many different kinds of bunions, and not all of them hurt. Some patients insist that a bunion developed "overnight," as a result of wearing a particularly uncomfortable pair of shoes, but that's impossible. The sudden discovery of a bunion simply means that you've finally noticed a protuberance that's been expanding slowly over a period of years—either because the area has started to hurt or because you have encased the bunion in a very tight pair of new shoes.

Your bunion won't necessarily become large enough or inflamed enough to require surgical removal. Many people have small bunions that appear at the side or on the top of the big toe in their early thirties, but these don't always grow big enough to cause a real problem. A switch to shoes with a wide, roomy toebox may remove the irritation not only from the bunion itself but also from painful calluses that form on the metatarsal heads.

If the bunion does continue to grow, you are apt to develop a condition called *hallux abducto valgus*, in which the big toe is pulled further and further out of line in toward your second toe. (*Hallux* means "great toe," *abducto* means "outward," and *valgus* signifies an abnormal twisting over.) In the most severe cases, the big toe is so misshapen that the nail is scrunched sideways against the second toe and can't even be seen from above. Bunions and overpronation can form a vicious circle. Your bunion may have its origins in the tendency of your foot to roll too far inward, placing extra pressure on the first metatarsal joint. Then the bunion grows, encouraging further pronation.

As I've already indicated, hereditary foot structure—especially flat feet—predisposes some people toward bunions. These "inherited" bunions declare themselves early in life in both sexes, although studies suggest that even during the teen years, girls have twice as many bunions as boys. However, the prevalence of serious bunions rises dramatically in women with age, while it remains virtually the same for men in all age groups. When Michael J. Coughlin, M.D., a past president of the American Orthopaedic Foot and Ankle Society, surveyed his surgical practice over a fifteen-year period, he found that he had performed approximately eight times as many bunionectomies on women as on men around age sixty, the beginning of the peak decade for bunion surgery. International studies have shown that the incidence of bunions in societies where people generally walk barefoot or wear cloth rather than constricting leather shoes is roughly equal in men and women.

No intelligent woman can ignore the implications of these statistics. While sixty-year-old men aren't much more likely to have disabling bunions than twenty-year-old men, the incidence of bunion surgery in women at sixty is three times that of women at twenty. Clearly, we're doing something to inflame our preexisting bunions that men don't do. Open the closet that contains your shoes, and you'll see what that "something" is. If you already have a bunion and want to avoid becoming a surgical case, you need to get rid of shoes that hurt your forefoot and encourage the growth of bone deformations.

SYMPTOMS

It's important to remember that the symptoms of a bunion are progressive. You may never develop all of them, and you certainly won't develop all of them at once. Here's the usual progression:

■ A slight protuberance at the base of your big toe seems to be increasing in size. *This may not hurt at all.*

■ In addition to the bump, your big toe seems to be rolling over, forcing your other toes to overlap. You may develop ingrown toenails or a hammertoe (in which the joint bends upward) as a result of the pressure. The "hammer" usually appears on your second or third toe.

■ Painful calluses emerge under the second or third toe, or at the tip of the abnormally angled big toe.

■ You have tremendous problems finding shoes that don't hurt your bunion.

■ The area around the bunion, known as the bursal sac, regularly becomes inflamed and swollen, causing excruciating pain. The pain is far worse than that of a bunion unaccompanied by bursitis. How do you know if you have bursitis at your bunion site? Push down on the bump. If the area turns a whitish color when you press it, and then turns red when you release it, you probably do have a bursa. (There may actually be fluid in the bursal sac.) Bursas are frequently hot to the touch, and they—like the bunion itself—grow over time.

FROM MY FILES

I've performed thousands of successful bunion surgeries, and these procedures are particularly satisfying to me as a podiatrist because they lead to such a major improvement in the quality of my patients' lives. There is truly nothing as gratifying for a surgeon as the restoration of mobility to someone who, for years, hobbled around in pain and was unable to find an ordinary pair of shoes to cover her bunion. But surgery should be a last resort after other, noninvasive ways of controlling bunion pain have failed. When a patient comes to me with a small protuberance that isn't yet causing significant pain or toe deformities, my entire focus is on changing her biomechanics to impede the growth of the bunion and, we hope, avoid surgery down the road.

Kate, thirty-seven, was just such a patient. She was experiencing an unfamiliar ache in both big toes when she walked any distance. She wasn't aware that she had bunions, because they weren't especially obvious to the naked eye and weren't big enough to interfere with her choice of shoes. I could feel the change in the bone, but Kate didn't believe me until I showed her an X ray comparing her emerging bunion with an X ray of a foot with a normal big toe and metatarsal joint.

Kate's problem was a typical case of early-stage, age-related bunion progression. The heels of her shoes were unevenly worn down—a giveaway that she was overpronating and regularly shifting too much weight onto the forefoot at the base of the big toe. She had gone through two pregnancies in the previous five years, and her arches had flattened out slightly. I explained that she needed better arch support to discourage the shift of pressure to the area of the foot where her bunions were developing.

I suggested prescription orthotic inserts, but Kate—whose insurance plan didn't pay for orthotics—wanted to try less expensive over-the-counter inserts. (The cost of prescription orthotics ranges from approximately $250 to $500, depending on the materials used and the area of the country. If your doctor prescribes orthotics, check with your insurance company to determine whether you're covered.)

There's absolutely nothing lost by trying nonprescription inserts first. They work well for some people, and they work better the younger you are and the less acute your problem. But they didn't do much to help Kate. Her toe pain receded slightly but returned a few months later, and the bunions themselves were becoming visibly enlarged. She agreed, after a four-month trial, that it was time to try prescription orthotics and to take a close look at her choice of shoes.

On the surface, there was nothing wrong with Kate's shoes. A lawyer whose profession demands that she dress conservatively for meetings with clients and courtroom appearances, Kate had never worn the kind of sexy, spike-heeled shoes that intensify pain and encourage the growth of bunions. Her daytime shoe wardrobe consisted mainly of classic round-toed pumps, of soft leather or suede, with one-and-a-half- to two-inch heels. After work, she usually wore heavily padded athletic shoes. But when I felt Kate's toes inside her shoes, I realized that she was making a common female mistake—wearing shoes at least a half size too small.

Kate hadn't had her foot measured in a shoe store since she was a kid, and she was still wearing the size 6B that she had worn before her two pregnancies. In fact, she needed a 6 1/2, not only to take the pressure off her bunion but also because her entire forefoot had spread out. When Kate started wearing larger shoes, the pain in her toes disappeared almost instantly. Prescription orthotics placed her foot in a corrected position and discouraged the overpronation that had shifted extra weight toward the area of the bunion.

Four years have passed, Kate's feet are still pain-free, and there has been no significant enlargement of her bunions. She's still using the same pair of orthotics—a reasonable investment for four years of freedom from pain. Of course, I can't predict what will happen fifteen or twenty years from now—one unknown factor is weight gain—but Kate is active, is physically fit, and has made the minor adjustments that I recommend to everyone with a small, early-stage bunion. At this point (especially in view of the fact that neither of her parents has large bunions), I'd be very surprised if she ever turns into a surgical case. The key to Kate's successful outcome was the early action she took before her bunion became excruciatingly painful. If you walk around in pain for years without adjusting your footwear or consulting a podiatrist—as many people with bunions do—you greatly lessen your chances of getting rid of the pain without surgery.

Dina, forty-three, the owner of her own management consulting firm and a mother of two, is typical of patients who do need a bunionectomy (surgical bunion removal) in order to end their pain and fit into normal shoes. "I don't have time for this," was Dina's first response when I told her that her pain was bound to become more and more disabling if she didn't make room in her schedule to have the larger of her two bunions removed.

This is an understandable response from any patient, of whatever age or gender, but it's especially common among working mothers. Who has less time to take care of her own medical problems than a mom who's juggling a full-time job and the needs of small children? Dina's problems were compounded by the fact that she's divorced and her job requires frequent travel.

At the time she became my patient in 1994, Dina's only stress-reliever was jogging—and she'd pulled up lame after a two-mile run along the beach near the Miami hotel where she was staying on business. "At first I thought I'd broken my foot because it hurt so badly," she told me. When Dina realized that she could still put weight on her bad foot, she tried to tough it out for several months, cutting back (slightly) on her running and hoping that one day the pain would disappear as suddenly as it had appeared.

Dina was typical of patients who originally believed that their bunions developed "overnight." In fact, her left-foot bunion was so large by the time she came to see me that she could hardly stand to wear a closed-toe shoe over it. Her big toe was already twisted in the *hallux abducto valgus* position. And she also had frequent bouts of bursa inflammation: The extreme pain she felt in Florda was probably triggered by an acute attack of bursitis.

Because Dina was so reluctant to have surgery (not that anyone is thrilled by the prospect), I proposed that she get not only a second but a third opinion. She consulted two orthopedic surgeons, one of them specializing in athletic injuries. Both doctors also recommended surgery, and one told her he thought she would need to spend eight weeks in a cast or on crutches. She decided to have me perform the operation because I was far more optimistic about getting her back on her feet, without a hard cast, in a matter of days rather than weeks.

Surgical Options

There are several types of bunionectomies, and, to be perfectly honest, most of them sound very scary. While many of my patients' fears are unrealistic, it's important for them to know exactly what is involved in the procedures and what to expect during the recovery period.

■ *Simple Bunionectomy*

This is the least invasive procedure: Only the bump itself is removed, and some of the soft tissue is repaired. (Bunions also pull your ligaments and tendons out of their normal position.) The best candidates are patients whose big toe is still straight—in short, those who see a doctor long before the bunion has had a chance to deform the rest of the forefoot. But if there's already a significant deviation of your big toe, you're likely to develop a new bunion in the same location if you don't have the toe itself straightened surgically. That's why this procedure is not used for the vast majority of bunionectomies.

■ *Fractured Bone Bunionectomy*

Fractured bone bunionectomies (there are more than 100 variations) are exactly what they sound like: the surgeon gently fractures a bone or bones in order to remove your bunion and realign the forefoot for proper healing. In one version, both the big toe (hallux) and also a portion of the first metatarsal bone, are fractured and realigned. After your bunion has been removed, both toe bones are then reconfigured for healing in a straight position In another common procedure, the surgeon might fracture only the big toe and remove a small portion of the first metatarsal. In a third variant, your big toe is left alone and the surgical fractures are made only in the metatarsal bone. Everything depends on the size and location of your bunion, and your doctor may recommend one of many variations too numerous to describe in detail here. Any of these surgeries may involve the insertion of surgical pins (depending on how large the bunion was and the condition of the bone), but they're removed after four weeks.

If this procedure is recommended, don't automatically say "nothing doing." I urge you to take time to think it over and, if you have doubts, get a second opinion. You'll probably need six to ten weeks to recover from this surgery. But the outcome—in terms of pain relief and appearance—will be much more satisfactory than the results of a more limited bunion removal procedure that doesn't do anything about your crooked toe.

■ *Keller Bunionectomy* (Joint Replacement)

This procedure involves removal of a small portion of the bone or joint from the base of your big toe. I rarely recommend this operation for active people because it can result in a stiffening and shortening of the toe. Eventually, in view of the progress being made in joint replacement, there will probably be effective artificial toe joint replacements to improve mobility after this surgery. At this point, however, replacements for foot joints are still experimental. They do not have anything like the highly successful track record of hip and knee replacement surgeries.

After consulting with two other surgeons, Dina decided on a fractured bone bunionectomy procedure. Hers was a typical ambulatory operation, with the uncomplicated recovery most patients can anticipate if they're in good health and aren't overweight. Here's what to expect:

Day 1: In a doctor's office or ambulatory surgery facility, you are likely to receive either a local anesthetic injected into the surgical site or an intravenous anesthesia similar to that used in many dental surgeries. You won't feel any pain in either case, but local anesthesia leaves you fully conscious, while IV sedation renders you largely unaware during the procedure. In recent years, most of my patients have opted for IV sedation and I generally recommend it. However, there are people whose anxieties about "losing control" are so great that they want to be fully aware during surgery. For this minority, local nerve blocks are often the better choice.

Your surgeon will make a small incision (about one to two inches) and then use an instrument, called a surgical oscillating sword, to remove the bump. Then the bones can be manipulated into the proper position for healing. Because the incisions used in this procedure are small, and the electrical operating instruments so precise, postsurgical scarring is minimized.

Many bunionectomies are now performed in doctors' offices or ambulatory surgery facilities, but if you have diabetes or another systemic circulation-impairing disease, your doctor will probably recommend hospitalization regardless of which procedure you choose. Dina's surgery took about an hour, an average time for such procedures. Like many patients, she had the bunion removed on Friday in the hope of going back to work (in a cut-out shoe and on crutches) on Monday.

Days 2–4: Your doctor will probably give you crutches or a walker, with instructions to stay off your feet as much as possible. You'll also want to ice the foot frequently and keep it elevated. Dina returned to work on crutches the following Tuesday, but some patients need to stay off their feet for a week. How much postsurgical pain will you feel? That's a highly individual matter, but—although I always write a prescription for mild painkillers—most of my patients say they don't need anything stronger than over-the-counter medications like Tylenol. One of the most common misconceptions about bunion surgery is that it causes more pain than the bunion itself did.

That may have been true a generation ago, but it definitely isn't true today. Because electrical surgical instruments are so much more precise now, there's much less trauma to the soft tissue and nerve areas around the bone. I'd have to say that both the instruments and diagnostic tools (including MRIs to map soft tissue and ultrasound to check circulation) bear about the same relationship to the tools I used as an intern as today's compact personal computers bear to the huge office computers that took up entire floors of buildings in the 1960s.

Days 4–14: You'll be back at work and able to put some weight on your foot, but you'll still have to keep your weight-bearing activities to a minimum. A soft surgical shoe, strapped with Velcro, should enable you to move around comfortably. The surgical incision should be completely healed within fourteen days. Any stitches will then be removed. Until the sutures are taken out, you'll have to avoid getting your foot wet.

Since you won't be able to immerse the stitches in a bath, you'll probably want to take a shower while keeping the foot (protected by a plastic bag) out of the spray as much as possible. Warning: Be extremely careful while you're doing this, using a no-slip pad beneath your feet in the shower. It's better to feel grungy for two weeks than to fall and break a bone while you're waiting for your stitches to come out.

2–8 Weeks: If any internal surgical pins were used during your bunionectomy, they will be removed at this time in your podiatrist's office. During this period, you should be given special exercises, under the supervision of a physical therapist, to strengthen the muscles of your foot, ankle, and lower leg. I consider rehabilitative exercise a critical factor in successful recovery from bunion surgery. Any surgery—anywhere in the body—creates a weakness in the affected area during the healing period. With carefully supervised exercises, you can prevent muscle and tissue atrophy, and prepare yourself for more aggressive physical therapy after the initial period of healing is over. Six to eight weeks after the surgery, you should be able to return to wearing regular shoes, in soft materials that don't place pressure on the healing area. Exactly six weeks after her bunionectomy, Dina was able to wear attractive sandals—with an open front to accommodate the area where surgery had been performed—to a college graduation.

8 Weeks–6 Months: Your foot will probably feel perfectly normal when you walk, but you may still experience swelling and pain if you overdo. I recommend a continued program of supervised physical therapy, especially for patients like Dina who want to return to activities like running. The great danger during this period—especially for fitness enthusiasts—is overdoing and setting back the recovery process. When people have been suffering from a painful bunion for a long time, the end of the pain is such a relief that they frequently think they can do anything. Four to six months after surgery, you probably will be able to do everything you want. I say probably because recovery from all forms of surgery is a highly individual matter. But I've found that approximately 90 percent of my patients meet these recovery "deadlines."

Although you'll be back in regular shoes six to eight weeks after a bunionectomy, it's important not to return to the ill-fitting footwear that aggravated and encouraged the growth of your bunion before surgery. Many women are overjoyed because they can fit into high-heeled high-fashion shoes for the first time in years. That's fine for the occasional evening, but you should be extremely careful about what you wear every day. Soft materials—suede instead of stiff leather, for instance—and ample room in the forefoot are crucial.

Throw out any shoes, of whatever heel height, that come to a point in front. You don't want your bunion to return in five or ten years. Dina, like many women who've had successful bunion surgery, says she's become a master of "the invisible shoe shift." She keeps a pair of soft bedroom slippers underneath her desk, and she never leaves her office for a meeting with a client without carrying a pair of fitness shoes. "The high heels are for show," she says. "The minute the client and I shake hands and say good-bye, it's off with the heels and on with the walking shoes."

PREVENTION AND SELF-CARE

■ If your bunion is small and you're trying to live with it, over-the-counter moleskin pads or foam may alleviate the pressure if you also shift to larger, softer shoes.

■ If your feet hurt in shoes but you can't bear to part with them (the shoes, that is), a skilled shoe repair person may be able to stretch out the forefoot of your pumps. However, there's no real substitute for shoes that fit properly.

■ All of my recommendations for postsurgical shoe shifts apply just as strongly to people with bunions who are trying to avoid surgery.

■ Over-the-counter drugs containing ibuprofen or aspirin sometimes help bunion pain. If you're using these drugs on a regular basis and can't stand the pain without them, however, it's time to see a podiatrist.

■ If you suddenly find that you're in acute pain (and this always seems to happen on a Friday before a three-day weekend, when no medical help is available), apply ice packs to the area three or four times a day. You probably have an acutely inflamed bursa, and it's important to cool it down. Put your foot in a tub of ice and keep it there as long as you can stand it if packs don't bring down the swelling. Over-the-counter anti-inflammatories may also help. If you have a fever for more than twenty-four hours, see a doctor. Your bursal sac may be not only inflamed but also infected.

■ Here's another home remedy that I've found particularly helpful for bursitis attacks. Soak the area for fifteen minutes in a mixture of one cup of vinegar and a gallon of warm water.

■ Experiment with over-the-counter nonprescription inserts in your shoes. These don't correct overpronation, but they do provide cushioning that may make you feel more comfortable.

■ Wear socks that fit properly inside your athletic shoes. Too-loose socks are an extra source of irritation to an already inflamed area.

■ If you have frequent bursitis attacks in your toe joint, that's a definite sign that you need to consult a podiatrist. If you're scared because you think you might need surgery, remember that the larger the bunion gets, the more likely you are to need an operation to get rid of your pain.

6

Calluses

WHAT GOES WRONG?

Even though you may not like the way they look, ordinary calluses are basically good for you. These layers of dead, thickened skin are nature's way of protecting body parts that are expected to do a great deal of work and are exposed to constant friction and pressure. Gardeners, painters, and carpenters usually have calluses on their palms from constantly handling the tools of their trade. You'll see calluses on the inside of your middle finger (from holding a pen), your elbows (from leaning on desks and tables), and, above all, on the outside of your big toes, your heels, and the balls of your feet. Runners invariably develop extraordinarily thick calluses—a first line of defense against the greatly increased pressure they place on their feet.

Normal calluses don't hurt: Your body builds up the skin in a highly successful effort to protect bones in areas with a minimal cushion of natural fat. (It's obvious why we don't need calluses on our bottoms.) Most men don't give a second thought to painless calluses, but women sometimes want them removed so that their feet will have a softer, smoother look in summer sandals. While it's fine to smooth the skin by moisturizing it and using a pumice stone, it's not medically necessary to get rid of such calluses. If you regularly engage in any form of weight-bearing exercise or if you spend a good deal of time on your feet, you probably need the extra cushioning.

There are two main causes of painful calluses. Sometimes, a callus develops around a wart or foreign body that eventually becomes infected. More commonly, a sore callus is the body's response to a biomechanical irregularity affecting your gait (often caused by a slight variation from the norm in the foot's bone structure).

SYMPTOMS

■ Pain when you walk. Calluses almost never hurt while you're resting.

■ Deep heel fissures—these may even be deep enough to bleed—on the outside of the callus.

■ Visible inflammation and/or heat that doesn't go away when you take the pressure off the callus. This is unusual and generally means that there's an infection caused by a foreign body trapped underneath. I've found many calluses encasing slivers of wood, shards of glass, or microscopic pieces of gravel. The calluses did their job too well, preventing the patient from realizing that her foot had absorbed a sharp microscopic invader. The obvious and simple solution: Remove the offending object and disinfect the immediate area.

Painful calluses caused by flawed biomechanics are more complicated to treat because they are the body's attempt to "even out" your walking surface. One example is the callus created by what podiatrists call a "dropped metatarsal." In this condition, one of the sesamoids (those eyeball-shaped bones behind your big toe) is lower than the other and you develop a thick, extraordinarily deep callus to level out your gait. In similar fashion, a callus almost always forms under the second metatarsal bone if your first metatarsal is too short. Still other calluses—often among the most painful—are associated with bunions and hammertoes.

The reason why these calluses hurt is that the body's adaptive strategy—creating formations of painless thick skin—doesn't work forever. Eventually, as the callus continues to grow and deepen, it impinges on healthy tissue, which *can* feel pain. Extremely deep calluses put pressure on the nerves and blood vessels, and that's when you begin to hurt, sometimes excruciatingly.

If the sore callus is simply one more secondary symptom of a serious bone, joint, or toe problem, it won't go away until you deal with the underlying medical condition. If you have a severely enlarged and inflamed bunion, for instance, the painful adjacent calluses will continue to cause trouble until the bunion itself is surgically corrected.

More commonly, though, the biomechanical problems that lead to calluses (including those related to early-stage bunions) can be corrected with relative ease. Sore calluses develop most frequently on the balls of the feet, often as the result of overpronation if you have low arches. Extremely high arches, too, can help produce these calluses. In these cases, noninvasive podiatric treatment, which may include custom-fitted orthotics, is highly effective.

FROM MY FILES

When I first saw Ariane, a former professional dancer and actress in her early forties, she had developed painful calluses (along with corns) for the first time in her life. Like many people in their forties, she was losing some of the fatty cushion on the soles of her feet, and she also had unusually dry, thinning skin. When Ariane walked into my office wearing ballerina flats with paper-thin soles, I knew that her shoes were also contributing to her problem.

It's important for women to realize that extremely flat shoes, as well as extremely high heels, play a significant role in many painful foot conditions. Women who regularly wear heels higher than two inches, and who keep their dressy shoes on all day, are apt to develop extrathick calluses on the balls of their feet because their shoes are encouraging excessive weight shift onto the metatarsal bones. Ariane's ballerina flats, by contrast, encouraged excess callus formation because they didn't provide enough cushioning for the entire soles of her feet.

I suggested that Ariane shift to pumps with one-inch heels in order to take the pressure off all of her calluses. I've made the same suggestion in reverse to women whose calluses are the result of a full-time passion for high heels. Whatever shoes you prefer, you'll be doing your feet a favor if you vary your footwear, and your heel height, from day to day and several times during each day. By changing shoes, you discourage the excess callus buildup that occurs when your foot strikes the ground in exactly the same place all the time.

Over a period of several weeks, I got rid of Ariane's painful calluses by moisturizing and debriding them (paring them down) with a sterile surgical blade. I call this a "medical pedicure," since it not only relieves pain but also improves the appearance of heavily callused feet. (As I've already indicated, I *don't* recommend the removal of calluses purely for the sake of appearance if they aren't bothering you.)

GETTING A PEDICURE

I'm well aware that many women have long relied on commercial beauty parlors and nail-care salons for what they consider minor repair work like callus removal. This is a mistake—and I'm not saying that because I want the work. I frequently see the results of my patients' encounters with nonsterile instruments and whirlpool basins in nail parlors. Heel fissures crack open and bleed because a manicurist accidentally dug into healthy tissue while she was trying to pare away a callus. Fungus nails (caused by highly contagious organisms) suddenly emerge after an encounter with a contaminated water-filled basin. And there's always the possibility of contracting a truly serious infection, like hepatitis, in a setting where you simply can't be sure how clean the instruments, lotions, ceramic basins, and even the hands of the staff really are.

Feel free to pamper yourself with a pedicure as long as you bring your own instruments (and disinfectant for the basin), but please don't turn over any procedure that involves a sharp instrument to anyone but a medical professional. When calluses are already painful and inflamed, it can be difficult for anyone but a podiatrist to know where the dead skin ends and healthy tissue begins. Most health insurance plans will reimburse you for routine podiatric procedures; check with your insurance company if you have any doubt.

Calluses like Ariane's will re-form from time to time but can be pared down before they cause any pain. Like most of my patients who've had their originally painful calluses removed, Ariane is now able to keep her feet comfortable through self-care at home. For people with extremely dry, thinning skin, moisturizing is not a cosmetic luxury but a medical necessity. I see Ariane about once every three months, when she comes in to have excess skin pared away before it becomes a problem.

The Europeel

There's a new and wonderful high-tech procedure, called the Europeel, that I've used with great success to remove extremely tough calluses. This is basically a high-powered vaccum pump in reverse; it pushes aluminum oxide crystals into the callused skin and softens it. In many cases, this procedure is superior to debriding with a blade precisely because there isn't any cutting involved. It softens callused skin evenly, so there's no danger of a less-than-smooth result on the bottom of the foot. I expect that this procedure will become available in many more podiatric offices during the next few years. The gentleness of the process is particularly important for high-impact exercisers who need to maintain some of their callus formation for protection but want to avoid the kind of excessive buildup that hurts.

PREVENTION AND SELF-CARE

- If your callus isn't consistently painful but causes you occasional discomfort, an ordinary moleskin pad from the drugstore may give you instant relief.
- Think about your footwear habits. Are you wearing the same shoes—or shoes of the same heel height—for eight, ten, twelve hours a day every day? Try switching shoes back and forth, and, if that doesn't help, experiment with nonprescription heel and metatarsal pads available in athletic footwear stores and pharmacies. They won't hurt you and may help.
- If your calluses are caused by a rapid loss of fatty tissue under the ball of your foot, or a bone deformity, your podiatrist may recommend a prescription orthotic device—custom shoe

inserts made from a cast of your foot. Most patients want to try over-the-counter inserts first, because they're much less expensive than the custom variety. One warning: If you're experimenting with an over-the-counter insert and feel unaccustomed pain in your lower back, knee, or ankle, stop using the product immediately and consult your podiatrist. You don't want to get rid of callus pain by subjecting your joints to extra stress.

If you're not sure which of the many over-the-counter inserts are likely to help you—the vast array of products can be utterly confusing—buy several samples and ask your podatrist to take a look at them. You can return the ones that aren't appropriate (if you haven't opened the package).

■ Many people try to remove painful calluses with commercial pads in which the active ingredient is salicylic acid. I don't recommend this, because salicylic acid is a caustic ingredient that may harm the surrounding skin. As I've indicated, truly painful calluses are almost always the result of faulty biomechanics, and what you need to do is figure out a way to take the pressure off the spot. Remove a callus with acid, and it will soon return if you haven't taken care of the biomechanical problem.

■ Soak your callused feet in warm water for about fifteen minutes every night. Use a pumice stone or abrasive brush, followed by a moisturizer before bed. All moisturizers—cosmetic ads laying claim to "secret ingredients" notwithstanding—contain basically the same ingredients: vegetable oils, lanolin, "wool fat" (especially soothing oil products from sheep), collagen, and, of course, herbs and flowers that create a distinctive scent. Medically speaking, there's little difference among low-cost generic brands, medium-priced mass-market cosmetics, and expensive creams and lotions beautifully packaged and sold in high-end department stores.

If your calluses are extremely thick, try a dry skin product with an ingredient called urea, which, used over a period of weeks, softens the skin buildup so that you can get rid of the dead cells with a brush or pumice stone. Look for products with a urea content of 20 percent. Caution: Do not apply either urea cream or non-urea cosmetic lotions to calluses with open, inflamed fissures. This may cause further inflammation or promote bacterial infection. Keep a sterile pad over the fissure until it closes and then start applying cream. All lotions and creams work better if you cover your feet with clean white socks before going to bed. And never use moisturizer on unwashed feet: You simply seal in bacteria. In my opinion, the most effective moisturizer of all—and the cheapest—is petroleum jelly.

■ I'm a big believer in home remedies for calluses, and here are two of my favorites:

—Dilute a chamomile tea bag with two quarts of warm water and soak for fifteen minutes. The chamomile will stain your feet, but the discoloration can easily be washed away in cool water. You'll find that the calluses are much softer and more amenable to reduction.

—Make a paste of 1 cup of kosher salt, 8 tablespoons of mineral oil, 1/2 cup of Epsom salts, and 1 tablespoon of baking soda. Apply the paste to all of the most callused spots on your foot, put the entire foot into a plastic bag, and wrap a warm towel around everything. Sit still for ten minutes, unwrap your foot, and use a pumice stone on it. You'll be amazed at how quickly the dead skin falls away.

■ Whatever you do, don't try to pare down your own callus with a sharp instrument. When you attempt to do the job in a contorted position—and you can't "operate" on yourself without twisting your body into a pretzel—you won't know when to stop. You'll realize you've gone too far only when you hit live nerve endings and blood starts to spurt. I've treated many of these self-inflicted wounds, and they often have to be bandaged for weeks because they're in such sensitive areas.

A SPECIAL WARNING . . .

Never attempt to treat your own calluses, even with pumice stones and lotions, if you have been diagnosed with a disease impairing circulation to your hands and feet. These include diabetes and rheumatoid arthritis, but you should ask your doctor about foot care if you've ever been told that you have any condition affecting your vascular system. Impaired circulation renders you especially vulnerable to infections that gain entry through fissures in your feet.

7

Corns and Blisters

WHAT GOES WRONG?

Corns and blisters are the common colds of foot pain. And, like the common cold, they usually stop bothering you if you treat them at home with the podiatric equivalent of chicken soup.

Corns, like calluses, are protective areas of thickened skin that develop in response to friction. They may appear on top of, at the tips of, or between the toes, and on the outside portion of the little toe. Corns are yellowish in color, and they turn red when they're inflamed. The central core of your corn descends in a point into your flesh, killing all of the normal tissue it encounters. These are called hard corns, in contrast to the soft corns that may form between toes. Soft corns look and feel more like blisters; the perspiration between your toes prevents them from hardening.

Blisters are fluid-filled sacs that form between the top layers of skin. Like corns, they're almost always a response to irritating shoes. Unlike corns, they don't extend downward into your flesh. Blisters often cause more intense short-term pain than corns. They're particularly annoying to people who maintain a regular athletic or exercise routine, because there's really nothing to do about a blister except stay off it until the skin heals. Major-league pitchers miss starts, and ballet dancers important performances, because they're nursing brand-new blisters.

SYMPTOMS

■ You obviously won't have any trouble recognizing ordinary corns (they even look like the cartoon depictions of corns in television commercials for over-the-counter remedies). Most corns, particularly those on your vulnerable little toe, grow larger over time—whether or not they hurt—in response to pressure from shoes.

■ If your corn suddenly becomes extremely sore and hot to the touch, your pain may be caused by a swollen bursa, the fluid-filled sac between the bone and the corn. Bursas protect all of the joints in your body, and they swell up in response to extra pressure.

■ Blisters are soft, and you always see a whitish sac, filled with fluid, near the surface. If the blister becomes extremely irritated, the sac may fill up with blood. On occasion, a hard corn and a soft blister may be so close to each other that it's difficult to tell them apart.

PREVENTION AND SELF-CARE

■ For temporary relief of pain of a corn caused by an inflamed bursa, soak your feet in a solution of warm water and Epsom salts, which you can buy in any drugstore. You may find newer and more expensive preparations to deal with this pain, but you won't find any that work better than the salts your grandmother used.

Soaking for at least an hour dramatically reduces the soreness by bringing down the swelling (that's how you know there was bursal inflammation beneath the hard corn). If you can soak for more than an hour in a relaxing hot tub, that's even better. Usually, you realize that an attack of bursa pain followed some change in your routine—most likely, wearing a stiff pair of new shoes for several hours. If you put those shoes back on again, the sac will swell up once more in far less time than it took to bring down the inflammation by soaking.

■ When you have a painful blister and can see the fluid underneath the surface of the skin, wash the area gently with soap and water and use some alcohol (or Betadine solution) to disinfect it. Then puncture the surface very carefully with a disinfected sharp instrument and let the fluid out. Apply a topical over-the-counter antibiotic cream and cover with a sterile pad. Be extremely careful about taking sanitary precautions, because blisters can easily become infected after you've opened them up.

■ To discourage a recurrence of the blister, try putting a piece of moleskin or lambswool on the affected area. Rubbing these sensitive areas with petroleum jelly, or powdering them, can help reduce friction. If you developed a blister after increasing or changing your athletic activity, ill-fitting, loose socks or the wrong athletic shoes could be responsible.

■ If you're like everyone else, you've probably spent a small fortune on over-the-counter corn remedies. All of these corn pads, like callus pads, contain salicylic acid. And while they often reduce the size of your corn if you use them according to the instructions on the package, there's always a danger of eating away healthy tissue and causing yourself additional pain.

Also, salicylic acid can sometimes produce blisters—so you wind up with a double inflammation at the site of your corn. If you want to reduce the size of your corn at home, I recommend a soak in Epsom salts first, followed by moisturizing cream. Cover the area with a plastic wrap for at least fifteen minutes and then use a pumice stone. It's just as risky to use sharp instruments on your corns as it is to perform amateur surgery on calluses. If you want to get rid of most of the lump in a short period, leave the paring to a podiatrist.

And remember: Whatever method you use to get rid of your corn, the bump will return if you continue to wear shoes that irritate the area. Warning: Never use a salicylic acid pad on an inflamed corn.

■ If you repeatedly develop new blisters, or you have chronic pain from corns and bursal flare-ups, your shoes probably don't fit properly. They're either too narrow or too short or both. You may also need differently cut athletic shoes for different activities, because shoes that don't cause blisters when you run may hit you in a different spot when you're playing tennis.

A SPECIAL TIP FOR WOMEN . . .

Sandals with extremely narrow straps across the toes—even if the shoes themselves are the right size—are particularly likely to cause blisters.

8

Fallen Arches, Flat Feet, and Plantar Fasciitis

WHAT GOES WRONG?

If you're one of a minority of children who really were born with "flat feet," you've probably been hearing the term since you were old enough to understand what your pediatrician was saying. You inherited a bone structure with a very low arch that causes your foot to lie flat against the ground when standing. It's easy to tell the difference between a flat and a normal arch when you're walking barefoot near the edge of the ocean. A normal arch produces a "divided" footprint, with deep impressions where your heel and forefoot strike the ground, separated by a lighter imprint (or no imprint at all) that reveals the flexing upward of the metatarsal arch during your gait cycle.

The gap in the footprint means that your arch barely grazed the ground—or never touched it at all! (Of course, we're not aware of this flexion when we walk; it *feels* as if the entire foot is touching ground.) But if you have truly flat feet, you'll see one undivided print, visual evidence that your arch is spreading out and touching ground with every step.

For most of us, flat feet aren't born but are made through the wear and tear of a lifetime of walking. As the soft tissues in the foot react to the pressure they've absorbed over time, they sag—and so does the arch. The clear two-part footprint of a twenty-five-year-old starts to blur into one print in the forties. For fitness enthusiasts who've put more miles on their feet through exercise, arches may begin to sag long before midlife. The vital plantar fascia ligament, which stretches from the heel to the big toe, may become badly inflamed as it loses its resiliency and hits the ground with every step. This is called plantar fasciitis.

Many patients prefer to be diagnosed with plantar fasciitis rather than the more mundane fallen arches. Whatever you call it—even when the plantar fascia inflammation is caused by athletic overexertion—fallen arches and plantar fasciitis generally go together. In people over thirty, they're part of the same aging process. "You mean I have what my grandmother was always complaining about?" wailed a forty-five-year-old lawyer whose arches had been killing him since he started running three miles a day. I had to tell him yes.

Many young adults with flat feet have no trouble at all, although arch pain can develop at any age when an inactive person suddenly begins an exercise program. In the late thirties and forties, early arthritic changes in the bones of the midfoot may combine with sagging ligaments to affect pronation, the way your weight shifts from the back to the front of your foot as you walk. In normal pronation, your foot strikes the ground heel first, rolling forward toward the toes, with the arch dipping and then curving upward as each step is completed. When the arch dips too much, hitting the ground with each step, and your foot rolls too far inward, you're walking with what podiatrists call overpronation. And that can create a host of painful problems, as your foot and the rest of your body try to compensate for the abnormal distribution of pressure.

SYMPTOMS

■ Your arch may ache at any time, but the pain always worsens during and after exercise. The arch area feels tender when you press on it. When you get out of bed in the morning, your feet hurt even more than they do at the end of the day.

■ Heel pain.

■ The inside of your ankle swells. This happens because your ankle is working harder to compensate for the loss of flexibility in your foot. The outside of the ankle may hurt too, but the inside becomes involved first.

■ The back of your ankle feels tight and sore. If your Achilles tendon is too tight—and that's often the case in adults over thirty—it may become highly inflamed by the additional stress placed on the ankle.

■ If you have a bunion, it hurts more and may become visibly inflamed. Sometimes, you may even notice a bunion—because it's getting bigger—that you never knew you had. That's because your feet are overpronating—shifting more weight toward the toe—in an effort to spare your aching arches. Your big toe joint is feeling the pressure.

FROM MY FILES

Susanna, at twenty-nine, is one of the younger patients I've treated for arch pain. She doesn't have truly flat feet, but her arches couldn't handle a high-impact step aerobics class she'd begun taking at her health club. Three weeks after she started the aerobics—which she loved—she stepped out of bed in the morning and literally screamed when her feet hit the floor. I told her to take a cab to my office immediately, because she was in tears on the phone.

The acute pain of a badly strained plantar fascia ligament is hard to describe to anyone who hasn't experienced it. Like Susanna, most people going through their first bout of plantar fasciitis are terrified that they've torn or broken something inside their foot. It's hard for anyone to imagine that a mere *strain*—an overstretched ligament and a sagging arch—could hurt so much. People who are young, healthy, active, and of normal weight—as Susanna was—simply can't imagine that anything so painful could go wrong with their feet.

Susanna was relatively easy to treat because she sought help right away instead of trying to walk around while hoping that the pain would magically disappear.

Like most people, Susanna didn't develop arch pain in both feet at the same time. Just as we all have one foot slightly larger than the other, we all tend to put more weight on one foot. I gave her a whirlpool treatment to ease the tightness and soreness, strapped her right foot and ankle tightly in an elastic bandage—which gave her some relief immediately—and recommended that she stay off her feet as much as possible for forty-eight hours. I also told her to ice the sole of her foot and her ankle (which was slightly swollen on the inside).

With Susanna's pain greatly eased after two days, I showed her simple exercises to stretch out her calf muscles and heel cord first thing in the morning and before her aerobics class (see Appendix B: "Exercises"). These stretches, which take no more than ten minutes, are the key to overcoming many kinds of foot pain, including plantar fasciitis. If the heel cord is too tight, the plantar fascia ligament must work much harder every time the foot flexes. Eventually—with or without classic "flat feet"—this creates strain and pain in the arch. Everyone over thirty should do these stretches at least twice a day, and they make a perfect warm-up for runners and fitness walkers.

To prevent a recurrence, Susanna also had to change her shoes. She generally wore ballerina flats, with no heels and almost no cushioning on the inner or outer soles, exactly the wrong shoe for someone with sore arches. Because the adverse effects of spike heels are well known, many women assume that the best shoe for their feet is totally flat. In fact, the best shoe is one with a heel of one to one and a half inches, which creates an arch without putting your foot into the unnatural position created by spike heels. Patients like Susanna often experience an immediate cessation of arch pain when they shift from ballerina flats to a one-inch heel. (In the acute stage of plantar fasciitis, I recommend that patients never walk barefoot around the house but always put on a heeled shoe or slipper.) I also had Susanna insert a small, nonrescription metatarsal pad in all of her shoes, including those she used for exercise.

One of Susanna's main goals was to resume her step aerobics, but I recommended that she work her feet back into shape with a lower-impact class. She started taking low-impact aerobics a month after her first visit to me (by which time she'd been pain-free for two weeks). Three months later, she resumed the step aerobics. With cushioning in the arch of her shoe and stretches before exercise, she's had no recurrence.

Susanna's pain was simple to remedy because she was young, was in good shape, had none of the bony deformities that so often accompany fallen arches in older adults, and was treated early in the cycle. For many patients, though, it can take months rather than weeks to alleviate severe pain in the arches.

Daniel, a forty-five-year-old city government administrator, was a much more difficult case. For whatever reason (he couldn't explain it), Daniel had put on thirty pounds in the six months before he came to see me. Like many men, he had waited longer to seek medical help for his pain than women do. During our first consultation, he said he'd been experiencing soreness only for a few weeks, but I suspected that he'd been minimizing his pain—toughing it out—for several months. He had come to my office straight from a hospital emergency room, an indicator of the severity of his pain on that day. After determining that he had no broken bones, the emergency room doctor referred Daniel to me.

Unlike Susanna, Daniel was in so much pain that an immediate anti-inflammatory injection was indicated. I use both anti-inflammatory steroids and painkillers like Xylocaine in these cases: It's impossible to correct the biomechanics of a patient like Daniel while the area is so acutely inflamed.

However—and I can't stress this enough—anti-inflammatory injections should be used only as a short-term measure. I never give a patient more than three injections (usually over a three-week period). If the pain isn't significantly reduced by then, it's time for more sophisticated diagnostic testing—an MRI (magnetic resonance imaging) to rule out soft-tissue tears that can't be detected by conventional X rays and an ultrasound to make sure that there's no problem with blood circulation. More often than not, these tests confirm that there's no larger problem but that the patient has an unusually severe case of plantar fasciitis in conjunction with fallen arches.

Not all of my colleagues agree with me, but I think it's a red flag if a doctor continues to administer regular anti-inflammatory injections after a month—and you continue in agony after the drug wears off. What's wrong with these shots if they make you feel better? The answer is that they're only masking your symptoms without treating the underlying cause: The false sense of security produced by steroid relief may lead you to injure your foot further because you can't feel the warning transmitted by pain. We see this all the time with professional athletes, who are given steroid shots for supposedly minor injuries so that they can "play through the pain" for the benefit of their teams and the team owners' profits. Suddenly, what was originally described as a "strain" in the sports pages becomes a "rupture"—and the athlete needs surgery for what may be a career-ending injury. If he had rested for six weeks instead of continuing to play with steroid-suppressed pain, the strain might not have turned into a rupture. The same principle applies to nonathletes.

After three steroid injections, Daniel was still in considerable (though somewhat reduced) pain, and I prescribed nonsteroidal oral anti-inflammatory drugs to control his symptoms while he began a physical therapy regimen. The therapy included mild stretching exercises and electrogalvanic stimulation, which breaks up pain by increasing circulation to the foot. I also cast Daniel's feet for prescription orthotic devices, which were absolutely necessary because he was overweight. (The nonprescription metatarsal pads that worked so well for Susanna would have done nothing for Daniel.)

Daniel's condition did not respond to the orthotics at first. More than two months had passed, and although his pain wasn't as acute as it had been at the beginning of treatment, he couldn't walk without significant soreness. At one point, I thought I was going to have to put Daniel on crutches—something I try to avoid because it can lead to muscle atrophy.

This was a frustrating period for me and for my patient. As a doctor, my first priority is to relieve pain as quickly as possible; my second is to help the patient regain mobility. Daniel was still in considerable pain, and he wasn't able to walk more than a block without feeling worse. It was clear that the real cause of this acute episode was Daniel's weight gain, and I told him I felt certain that he would begin to see real improvement as soon as he started to lose the weight.

Talking to patients about their weight is always a delicate matter. Since I used to be overweight myself, I know how hard it can be, when you're hurting, to hear someone tell you that too much food—one of the few things that can take your mind off pain—is part of your problem. Yet as a doctor, I know that weight gain is one of the major contributors to arch pain in people over forty. If you were born with flat feet, extra weight may turn them from a manageable annoyance into a potential surgical case. And if you have the more common age-related version of sagging arches and plantar fasciitis, you hurt more and have more frequent recurrences with every additional pound.

I never urge patients like Daniel to begin a crash diet that will make them feel starved (and, inevitably, depressed when whatever they lose comes back because they can't stick to the plan). Instead, I suggest that they try for a moderate weight loss—a pound a week is fine—to help them understand what a small decrease in weight can do for their feet.

When Daniel started losing weight, about three months after he began treatment, he began to feel better almost from day one (perhaps because he was taking charge of something he could control). As soon as he'd lost five pounds, his feet began to feel better, and he started to increase the length of his daily walks. Today, Daniel, like many non-car-owning New Yorkers, walks almost everywhere—and he's lost twenty-five pounds. Because his episode was so severe and of such long duration, I've advised Daniel to wear orthotic inserts and fitness shoes rather than business shoes if he's walking more than a few blocks. Of course, that's the same advice I give women about high heels.

FURTHER MEDICAL AND SURGICAL OPTIONS

Susanna's and Daniel's cases illustrate the most common forms of medical treatment for ordinary cases of fallen arches and plantar fasciitis. In neither case—although Daniel had particularly severe pain—was the arch pain accompanied by a rupture of the Achilles tendon or the tendon in back of the shin bone (posterial tibial tendon). Depending on the severity of rupture, surgery is sometimes recommended in these cases.

Operations to repair ruptured tendons are all complicated and require a recovery period lasting several months.

Surgery should be uncommon, but is sometimes unavoidable, when an injury associated with flat feet is the result of a long-standing bone deformity or recent severe trauma. In most cases, though, conservative, noninvasive methods should be given a chance for months—and should be tried again if there's a recurrence—before surgery is contemplated. You should get a second opinion, and all reputable surgeons—whether they are podiatrists or M.D. orthopedists—will encourage you to do so.

One operation that's also uncommon is performed in severe, intractable cases of plantar fasciitis. It's called an endoscopic plantar fasciotomy release, a procedure that detaches the fascia ligament from the heel bone, preventing it from pulling on the bone and causing pain. This is accomplished by inserting a delicate microsurgical instrument through two tiny incisions. It is an outpatient procedure performed under local anesthesia. When I began to practice as a surgeon, this procedure was extremely rare because it could be performed only by cutting the foot open, a traumatic surgery that was likely to cause more pain than it cured. Only with the aid of computer imaging—the endoscope serves as a telescope into the body to guide the surgeon—has it become possible to release the ligament without making a major incision. Although I've had wonderful results with this procedure in patients who haven't been helped in any other way, it *is* surgery and not to be taken lightly. I'd want to try at least nine months of noninvasive therapy before contemplating the operation.

Bunion removal (see Chapter 5, "Bunions") is one of the most common surgeries performed to correct deformities related to fallen arches. Fallen arches don't always cause bunions, but they do aggravate them. Combine sagging arches with the wrong shoes, and you're setting yourself up for trouble. People born with flat feet often develop bunions quite early in life, but many people who never had bunions in their twenties and thirties develop them as their feet flatten out in their forties and fifties.

To discourage a recurrence of bunions after surgical removal, I recommend stretching exercises, a change of footwear, and custom-fitted orthotic inserts—in short, the self-care regimen followed by both Susanna and Daniel. If you don't take care of your sore arches, you may fall into a perpetual cycle of renewed pain and bunion development, followed by still more surgery.

PREVENTION AND SELF-CARE

- Do the stretching exercises I've suggested (your doctor or physical therapist may recommend additional ones) at least twice a day, especially after you get out of bed and before you exercise. These are designed specifically to stretch out your heel cord (Achilles tendon), the muscles of your lower leg, and the plantar fascia ligament. If you can't or won't make the time to do all of these exercises, spend at least ten minutes on them.
- For walking, women should wear shoes with a one-inch heel, or padded athletic shoes with an inner arch, in preference to flats or uncushioned tennis shoes. While men can't don one-inch heels (not in ordinary offices, at least), they can use a heel cushion or over-the-counter orthotic arch inside their shoes.
- Always wear well-constructed athletic shoes for exercise—from brisk walking to high-impact sports—and replace them regularly. Many of us tend to keep wearing our old shoes too long, and we don't realize that the cushioning has worn out. As a rule of thumb, if you exercise three or more times a week, replace your shoes every six months. If you exercise every day, or are a long-distance runner, you need new shoes more often.

■ If you're beginning any new form of exercise, start slowly. I've seen patients develop acute plantar fasciitis from an exertion as minimal as increasing their walks by a half mile a day, or upping the pace from a mile in forty-five minutes to a mile in thirty minutes. If you experience *any* pain in the arch of your foot, stop what you're doing. It's worth the money to consult a physical therapist or fitness trainer who will evaluate your condition and tell you whether you need to see a podiatrist.

■ If you're feeling mild soreness in your arch, over-the-counter pain relievers may offer temporary relief (though they don't always help). If you're exceeding the recommended dosage, or the pain persists for more than two weeks, consult a doctor. Prolonged use of over-the-counter products, like prolonged dependence on prescription drugs, may promote injury by masking your pain.

■ The most important thing many of us can do to banish arch pain is to lose excess weight. If you can't face the idea of a major diet, try losing just five pounds and see if it makes a difference. Patients have told me that the pain relief they experienced after losing the first five pounds gave them the incentive they needed to stay on a more ambitious diet.

■ If your arches feel sore whenever you walk—even if the pain is nagging rather than intense—see a podiatrist sooner rather than later. If you're aware of soreness that doesn't go away after, say, three weeks, it's time to seek medical attention. Levine's Law: For every week you walk around hurting, it takes two weeks of therapy for you to stop hurting.

A SPECIAL TIP FOR WOMEN...

If you've always worn extremely high-heeled shoes and want to switch to lower heels, do it in careful stages. Women who've worn high heels for most of their lives are apt to have artifically shortened Achilles tendons. If you switch from a three-inch to a one-inch heel overnight, the heel cord won't have enough give to accommodate the longer stretch. And if you strain the heel cord, you strain the plantar fascia ligament too—creating a self-induced case of plantar fasciitis. Give your heel cord time to adjust by taking down your shoe height no more than an inch—sometimes a half inch—about every two weeks. And do those stretching exercises morning, noon, and night while you're making the transition.

9

Hammertoes

WHAT GOES WRONG?

Many people assume that the oddly named hammertoe derives its name from an injury caused by a household hammer. There's a certain logic to this misconception: Drop a hammer on your toe, and you'll surely hurt it. In fact, the podiatric hammertoe is called that because it resembles similarly shaped hammers inside a piano. While piano hammers are essential to making beautiful music, a hammertoe is anything but beautiful.

Hammertoes are deformations of the inner middle joint (the proximal interphalangeal joint), usually in your second toe. Instead of lying flat, the joint becomes bent and twisted, with the tip of the toe pointing downward and a bump forming on top. At the beginning of this process, the joint is still soft, but it stiffens over time. As the tip of the toe points downward and the bump on the joint becomes larger, shoes become a constant irritation. If the twisted toe joint is the one near the tip instead of the middle, it's called a mallet toe.

Hereditary foot structure may place you at risk for hammertoes, just as it does for bunions. People with unusually high

84

arches, or an exceptionally long second toe, are more likely to develop hammertoes. Bunions and hammertoes, as we have seen, frequently go together: When your big toe is pushed into an unnatural position by a growing bunion, the second toe doesn't have enough room to lie flat.

Hammertoes may also be caused by traumatic injuries, particularly those involving dislocation of your metatarsal bones. In addition, certain circulatory and neurological diseases, such as diabetes and multiple sclerosis, contribute to joint deformities by restricting blood circulation to the toes.

Finally, ill-fitting shoes—no, you can't get away from them when you're talking about toe and joint pain—encourage the bending and stiffening of the "hammer." Like bunions, hammertoes are far more common in women than in men (a four-to-one ratio). If you habitually wear shoes that are too narrow or too short—that squeeze your forefoot into a point—you're at risk for hammertoes regardless of your hereditary foot structure. When there isn't enough space for your toes, they naturally curl up because they have nowhere else to go. This was the principle behind Chinese foot-binding, in which toes were curled under to such an extent that women were literally unable to walk. In an era when women can do and become whatever they want, it's hard to think about such painful "traditions." Yet in a less extreme way, some of us do the same thing to our feet. Sometimes, when a woman takes off a shoe with a stilettolike point, revealing a painful hammertoe underneath, I feel like crying. These were once the straight, beautiful, perfectly functioning toes of a baby, and now they will never be the same. I can perform surgery to correct hammertoes, but many of these deformities should never have been allowed to develop in the first place.

SYMPTOMS

■ The deformation of an advanced hammertoe is obvious: you may not know what to call it, but you know something is very wrong. It's most important to recognize the early symptoms of hammertoe, when the condition can be remedied without surgery. At this stage, the toe is still flexible. It lies flat when you're standing at rest, and you can straighten it out when it starts to curl. But you're able to see the toe curling under when you walk barefoot. You also feel some irritation inside your shoe, but you don't yet have an obvious bump or an extremely painful callus.

■ In the intermediate stage, a bump and growing callus become obvious on top of the toe. You may also develop problems like ingrown toenails as a result of the unnatural position and the rubbing of the toes against one another.

■ If your hammertoe symptoms are accompanied by cold feet, see a doctor immediately. As I've noted, a hammertoe may be a symptom of a systemic disease affecting your circulation. You need to identify and get treatment for the systemic problem before dealing with the hammertoe itself. Be particularly alert for early hammertoe symptoms if you have a family history of diabetes.

FROM MY FILES

Are you under the impression that all of my cases are success stories? It's as frustrating for the doctor as it is for the patient when proper treatment doesn't produce the desired results. Nina, a sixty-year-old fashion industry executive, is one of my favorite patients, so I was doubly frustrated when a routine in-office surgical procedure failed to fully correct the hammertoe that she'd been living with for ten years. What I think Nina's case really demonstrates is the importance of recognizing and pampering an early-stage hammertoe.

Nina's hammertoe was probably caused by a bunion that I removed surgically fifteen years ago, when she was in her mid-forties. Although bunion surgery was far more painful at that time than it is today, Nina had a swift recovery and outstanding results. Her bunion hasn't returned—one important measure of a successful bunionectomy—and even the scar from the incision is barely visible.

Even without the bunion, Nina's hammertoe continued to develop, eventually causing her pain even in extremely comfortable shoes. Although she used various pads and straps in an effort to keep her toe in a flatter position, nothing really worked. Finally, surgery was the only choice: Nina could hardly wear fuzzy bedroom slippers to meetings with clients in the fashion business.

There are two basic surgical procedures to correct hammertoes, and Nina's was the easier one. Her hammertoe was still flexible, meaning it hadn't fused rigidly in its deformed position. Nina's operation involved stretching the tendon along the top of her toe through a tiny incision so small that stitches weren't even needed. As the hammertoe progresses, the tendon stiffens along with the joint. But once the tendon is relaxed surgically, the toe usually lies flat and the patient can begin to walk normally again, without pain, after a recovery period of four to eight weeks. Like bunion surgery, hammertoe procedures are performed under local anesthetic.

Nina's pain was completely eliminated, but, for reasons that weren't apparent from X rays of her bones and an MRI of her soft tissue, the joint began to pop up again after several months. Every doctor knows that even the most frequently performed surgeries have variable results: Most patients recover from appendectomies with no complications, for example, but a small minority develop painful adhesions (unnatural unions of adjoining tissues created by surgical scarring). That's why no surgery, even under local anesthetic in an office, is ever truly routine. Although Nina has no pain, she doesn't like the way the toe looks, and—more important—her pain may return if the joint deformation progresses once again.

It's possible that Nina might have had a better result from a second, more complicated procedure to correct advanced hammertoes. This is called arthroplasty, and it involves actually removing the toe joint (also under local anesthesia). The patient ends up with a shorter toe and a large scar, but the pain is permanently eliminated—and the hammertoe can't come back because the joint is gone. In this procedure, a small surgical pin is usually placed in the toe and is removed in three to six weeks. Many of my patients, especially those who've been in pain for years, have been completely satisfied with this procedure. However, any removal of a joint is obviously more traumatic to the foot—and the entire body—than simply stretching a tendon through a tiny incision. Nina has decided to live with her less-than-perfect toe, using a special strap to keep it lying flat and always wearing roomy shoes. I agree with this decision, especially since she isn't in any pain. What Nina really has now is the equivalent of the early-stage hammertoe she started to develop many years ago.

PREVENTION AND SELF-CARE

■ If you have an early-stage hammertoe, take the pressure off with an over-the-counter pad and strap that protects the bump from chafing and keeps the toe in a relatively flat position.

■ Hammertoes, like bunions, are sometimes accompanied by bursal inflammation. That's probably the case if you have a sudden attack of excruciating pain in a toe that normally doesn't bother you too much. Treat an inflamed hammertoe as you would an inflamed bunion bursa, by icing the area and relieving the pressure with an open shoe. Over-the-counter anti-inflammatories may also help.

■ Pay particular attention to the length and the shape of the toebox in your shoes. If you change your footwear early enough in the progression of the hammertoe, you may never experience real pain. Square-toed pumps, which are frequently in fashion, are even better for your feet than round-toed shoes.

10

Heel Pain

WHAT GOES WRONG?

Most people develop some pain in their heels at some point in their lives. When our heels hurt, the soreness is usually attributable not to one but to many causes. Is your Achilles tendon too tight? As we've seen, that's the tendon that attaches your heel bone to the muscle enabling it to move. Is your plantar fascia ligament strained? That runs from your heel to the ball of your foot. Thinking about these connections among tissues, muscles, and bones, it's easy to see why the heel throbs when something isn't quite right with another part of the foot or ankle. As the old ditty goes, "The hip bone's connected to the thigh bone ... the thigh bone's connected to the knee bone. ..."

Heel pain becomes more common with aging. You may develop a heel spur—a bony protrusion caused by a growth of calcium that begins to project downward, touching your plantar fascia ligament. This spur is your body's reaction to additional pressure caused by sagging arches, weight gain, or a sudden increase in your exercise level. Many women experience heel pain for the first time during pregnancy. Biomechanically, what happens is that the heel spur stretches your arch beyond its accustomed length. The plantar fascia ligament is actually tearing slightly at the spot where it's attached to your heel. This may lead to internal bleeding and further calcification, in which new calcium deposits build up around the bony point of the spur and make it hurt even more.

But this biomechanically generated pain isn't necessarily accompanied by the emergence of a bony spur. Some people develop heel pain quite suddenly, as a result of increasing their activity level without paying sufficient attention to stretching out the Achilles tendon. Soreness may develop simply because the heel is losing some of its fatty cushion and the outer layer of skin is thinning, especially in women over forty. Even the common heel fissures resulting from dry skin can trigger a biomechanical pain cycle. If you're walking with an antalgic gait to avoid aggravating the fissures, not only your heel bone but the rest of your foot will develop unfamiliar aches.

Whatever the cause, heel pain is probably the most common reason people consult a podiatrist.

SYMPTOMS

■ Your heel (and sometimes the rest of your foot and ankle) hurts most when you get out of bed in the morning. That's because both the plantar fascia ligament and the Achilles tendon tighten up while you're sleeping. (This tendency of soft tissues to stiffen up at night increases with age.) When you get out of bed, the tissues haven't had time to warm up. If you have a heel spur, it touches the tip of your plantar fascia ligament for the first time in hours—and the ligament protests! Your foot and heel generally begin to feel better after you've been up and walking around for a few minutes.

■ You may have a visible clump of tissue at the back of your heel, just over the bone, called a pump bump by laymen and a Haglund deformity (after the doctor who named it) by podiatrists. This bump is much more common in women than men, and it's caused by shoes with hardened edges (sandal straps are a particular irritant) inflaming the back of the heel. Pump bumps and heel spurs develop independently, but if you happen to have both, you can't decide which part of your heel hurts most.

■ Tingling or numbness on the bottom of the foot. (This could mean that your heel pain is related to a circulatory problem.)

■ Thinning of the heel pad, so that you can easily feel the heel bone when you press on the area.

■ Shin splints often go together with heel soreness. The shin pain is caused by overpronation that makes your lower leg work harder to compensate for the excessive weight shift toward the ball of your foot.

FROM MY FILES

Sara, fifty-one, began complaining of acute heel pain soon after she began a program of aerobic walking, recommended by her internist as a way to help bring down her slightly elevated blood pressure without medication. Sara had never had any problems with her feet, and her doctor didn't warn her that a sudden increase in exercise—even exercise as seemingly effortless as walking—might create podiatric problems. By the time Sara hobbled into my office, she was suffering not only from heel pain in her right foot but also from an inflamed plantar fascia ligament, a common combination of symptoms. Like most people with this condition, Sara described getting out of bed in the morning as a form of torture. She made an appointment with me after badly stubbing her toe while hopping from her bed to the bathroom on her "good" foot.

Sara didn't understand why "just walking" could bring on the kind of pain she was feeling. She had always enjoyed walking, and she didn't see why her body should respond differently to a three-mile daily walk than to a one-mile stroll. In fact, she'd continued her fitness walking after her heel started to hurt because she couldn't believe that her new exercise routine was responsible. If she'd started running, she commented, she would have known enough to consult a trainer first.

My first prescription for Sara was rest and ice. I advised her to stop fitness walking altogether until the inflammation in her heel had subsided. An X ray showed that she did have a very small bone spur, but her pain was probably attributable to the combination of strains on the soft tissues of her foot and on her Achilles tendon. In this first acute stage of heel inflammation, one important commonsense measure is putting on a shoe with a heel before you get out of bed in the morning. This reduces the strain on both the Achilles tendon and the plantar fascia ligament.

I also cut a felt heel pad for Sara to wear inside all of her shoes. When her immediate pain eased, I cast her foot for orthotics, which I recommended she wear inside her athletic shoes during her fitness walks. I also gave Sara my usual Achilles tendon–stretching exercises to do at home and suggested that she consult a trainer before resuming her fitness walks. (The trainer, Sara later told me, had told her to increase her walking by no more than a half mile each week and to cut back immediately if she felt any renewed strain.) A year later, Sara is walking four miles a day without any problems. The key to preventing recurrences of heel pain is cutting back whenever you feel a slight strain.

If your pain persists, your podiatrist may also recommend ultrasound therapy or electrogalvanic stimulation treatments.

Surgical treatment, which is uncommon, though it may be necessary in some persistent and difficult cases, can include an endoscopic release of the plantar fascia ligament (see Chapter 8, "Fallen Arches, Flat Feet, and Plantar Fasciitis") or removal of the heel spur itself. Heel spur removal is particularly rare; in some instances, the surgeon simply shaves down the bone slightly instead of taking off the entire spur.

PREVENTION AND SELF-CARE

My recommendations in the prevention section for Chapter 8 are equally applicable to heel pain. When you understand that heel soreness, plantar fasciitis, and Achilles tendinitis are all related, you're well on your way to a lifetime of pain-free walking.

■ Do the calf muscle and heel cord stretching exercises in Appendix B (your doctor or physical therapist may recommend additional ones) at least twice a day, especially after you get out of bed and before you exercise.

■ As always, women should wear shoes with a one-inch heel, or padded athletic shoes with an inner arch, in preference to flats or uncushioned tennis shoes. Men can use a heel cushion or over-the-counter orthotic arch inside their shoes.

■ Always wear well-constructed athletic shoes for exercise—from brisk walking to high-impact sports—and replace them regularly.

■ If you're beginning any new form of exercise, start slowly. I've seen patients develop acute plantar fasciitis and heel pain from an exertion as minimal as increasing their walks by a half mile a day, or upping the pace from a mile in forty-five minutes to a mile in thirty minutes. If you experience *any* pain in the heel or arch of your foot, stop what you're doing. Consult a physical therapist or fitness trainer who will evaluate your condition and tell you whether you need to see a podiatrist.

■ The most important thing many of us can do to banish arch and heel pain is to lose excess weight. Patients tell me that the pain relief they experience after losing just five pounds gave them the incentive they needed to stay on a more ambitious diet.

■ Wear shoes with soles that have some "give." In recent years, there has been a proliferation of low-heeled fashionable shoes (often flat sandals) with completely rigid, highly lacquered soles that feel almost like a board to the touch. If there's no give at all, your heel hits an immovable object with every step.

■ Try gently stretching and flexing your feet in a sitting position before you get out of bed. A warm bath may also relax your muscles if you customarily have heel pain in the morning.

■ Don't become discouraged and give up your stretching exercises if a few weeks go by and you're still in pain. It took years for your heel cord to tighten up. There's no quick fix for this kind of pain, but if you persist in your exercises for several months, you will get results.

11

Ingrown Toenails and Other Common Nail Problems

WHAT GOES WRONG?

■ *Ingrown toenails* are among the most painful and preventable of foot complaints, whereby the toenail curves into the surrounding skin instead of growing straight outward. The skin responds by becoming inflamed, just as it would if you had picked up a tiny sliver of wood in the area. Eventually, if the pressure of the ingrown toenail on the surrounding skin isn't relieved, the area becomes infected. Sometimes, people create the infection themselves by picking at the skin around the nail.

You can treat a mildly inflamed ingrown toenail yourself by soaking it in warm water, washing it carefully, and trimming the nail straight across. (Many toenails start to grow inward because they've been cut on a curve.) Nonprescription antibiotic creams may help reduce the inflammation.

If the pain and redness don't go away in a few days, see a podiatrist. If the redness around the area is increasing, go immediately. The doctor will numb the nail at the base of your toe with a local anesthetic and remove the portion of the nail that's become trapped in the surrounding skin. *This does not hurt—you truly won't feel a thing.* The area might be slightly sore afterward, and you'll want to wear a soft or cut-out shoe for a day or two, but the pain will feel like nothing in comparison to the agony of a badly ingrown toenail. If your toenail was infected, your doctor may prescribe an antibiotic.

■ *Paronychia* is the medical term for a badly inflamed cuticle. This can be caused by rough manipulation of the skin during a pedicure or by compulsive behavior (similar to fingernail biting) in which you constantly pick at your cuticles. When the cuticle is inflamed, it can easily become infected.

You can treat this at home by soaking in a warm water and Betadine solution and applying a topical antibiotic. Like ingrown toenails, cuticle inflammation should be treated by a doctor if it doesn't go away in a day or two. Your podiatrist will take a laboratory culture to determine whether you need an antibiotic. You should never neglect an infected cuticle, because it can be a host for virulent bacteria, including dangerous staphyloccocus organisms. If your cuticle is infected, your podiatrist will drain it with a tiny incision under local anesthetic.

■ *Black-and-blue nails* are caused by a tiny hemorrhage beneath the nail bed, often the result of a bump you didn't even notice at the time. Sometimes these don't hurt, and there's no need to do anything about them. However, such discolorations may also be caused by a vitamin C deficiency or a more serious blood disorder. If I see significant discolorations of this nature, I always run a battery of blood tests just to make sure that there's no systemic problem. If you have persistent dark nail discoloration, be sure to mention it to your doctor during your regular checkup.

■ *Onychauxis* is an age-related condition in which the nail becomes extraordinarily thick (usually in people over sixty) and may form a "ram's horn" shape. If this bothers you, your podiatrist can file down the nail with a rotary burr.

■ Occasionally, the nail separates entirely from the nail bed. This condition is called *onychomadesis*, and it's particularly common in runners and other athletes whose nails may be traumatized by new running shoes. These shoes irritate the top of the nail, causing it to flake off. It may take up to six months for a new nail to grow in. You should use lambswool or other padding to protect the top of your nail during this period and be particularly careful about hygiene. When your nail bed is partially exposed, you're far more vulnerable to infection.

PREVENTION AND SELF-CARE

■ Pay attention to your toenails and fingernails because they're sensitive barometers of change in the rest of your body. Chronic arthritis, for example, can produce ridges in your nails. Any pronounced change in the color or consistency of your nails (not only the black-and-blue discoloration I've already mentioned) can be a sign of a nutritional deficiency. Know what your nails look like normally (constant use of nail polish and remover may cause permanent yellow discoloration) so that you can alert your doctor to any major change.

■ Cut your nails straight across and always use your own clean instruments. (See Chapter 21, "The Beautiful Foot," for tips on medically safe pedicures.) You can't be too careful about keeping your nails clean.

12

Morton's Neuroma

WHAT GOES WRONG?

Morton's neuroma (named, as usual, for the doctor who first classified it) is an acutely painful inflammation of the nerve sheath between two toes—usually the third and fourth, but sometimes the second and third. The origins of nerve pain in any area of the body can be quite mysterious, but it's fair to say that nerves always become inflamed because of some abnormal pressure, either from a traumatic injury or an activity that causes steady irritation. Some people develop nerve pain for no apparent reason after surgery, long after the surgical incision has healed. In some way, the operation must have traumatized the nerve, and when the nerve tried to regenerate, scar tissue formed and increased the painful pressure.

Morton's neuroma, like so many painful foot disorders, is seven times more common in women than in men. The incidence of neuroma rises sharply in women at age thirty, peaking (like bunions) at sixty. For men, the incidence of neuroma is the same at sixty as it is at twenty. Therefore, it's reasonable to conclude that women's shoes play a role in a disorder that is really the result of a nerve being squeezed beyond endurance. Dancers and runners of both sexes are particularly susceptible to neuroma.

SYMPTOMS

■ Sharp pain or burning under the affected toes, which may appear suddenly, with no warning, or intensify after a long period of persistent but less acute soreness.
■ When you press down on the affected area from above, the pain may be intolerable.
■ Numbness and tingling in the foot or toes.
■ Pain that persists even when you're not wearing shoes or walking.
■ In severe cases, the throbbing wakes you up at night.
■ Swelling and heat in the affected area.

FROM MY FILES

Josie, thirty-nine, had walked around with what she described as "tenderness" for nine months after she tramped around in stiff boots during a blizzard. When she came to me, she had all of the classic symptoms of a neuroma. She screamed when I pressed on the area between her third and fourth toes and said she couldn't "feel" her foot. Her leg sometimes felt numb, and the painful twinge between her toes even woke her up at night. I gave Josie an injection of cortisone mixed with novocaine, which provided her with some measure of relief. Her response to the injection confirmed my diagnosis of a neuroma. (A number of other conditions have similar symptoms but don't respond to local injections.) Over the course of the next month, I administered two more injections. These are temporary measures, which provide substantial pain relief to most patients but cannot be continued over a longer period.

The real treatment is to relieve the pressure that inflamed the nerve in the first place. Josie didn't believe there was any connection between her neuroma and her footwear because she rarely wore high heels. Her everyday shoes were conservatively cut loafers. But when I looked at Josie's shoes, I could see that they were narrower than her feet. And when I felt her toes inside her shoes when she stood up, I found that her loafers were a size too narrow and a half size too short.

Josie initially resisted my recommendation, pointing out that if she bought larger shoes, they would slip off her heel. This is a common problem that calls for creative solutions (usually a heel insert) from a skilled shoe repairman. Also, I recommended prescription orthotics to take the pressure off the forefoot, and these take up extra room in shoes. When Josie agreed to try larger shoes with orthotics, she improved steadily over time. That's usually the case with neuromas: The pain doesn't disappear overnight but diminishes gradually as the pressure is removed. In rare cases, surgery is recommended to remove the nerve. I perform such operations only when the pain is severe, intractable, and unresponsive to more conservative treatment over a long period. There's a good chance of complete pain relief if the nerve is totally removed and the patient wears proper footwear afterward—but if the patient doesn't change her footwear, new neuromas may appear.

Early diagnosis is really the key to nonsurgical success in treating neuromas. While some neuromas do seem to appear overnight in their acute stage, many more—like Josie's—start out with a persistent but initially bearable alternation of burning and numbness in the toes. You hurt in shoes but feel better when you take them off. Gradually, the pain worsens until it's there all the time, even when you're in bed at night.

PREVENTION AND SELF-CARE

■ Wearing shoes with a roomier toebox is the only way to take pressure off an existing neuroma. The guidelines I outline in Chapter 22, "Shoe Savvy," will help you choose shoes that discourage many of the painful conditions disproportionately seen in women.

■ Some vigorous weight-bearing activities, notably running, may set off a neuroma. If possible, temporarily discontinue the activity and see a doctor or trainer for advice on modifying your exercise program—and possibly changing your shoes—to avoid future problems.

13

Nail Fungus

WHAT GOES WRONG?

Nail funguses are highly contagious infections that are easy to acquire and difficult to get rid of. Unlike so many foot conditions, nail fungus is more common among men than women, probably because more men spend time in the moist, warm environment of locker rooms, which provides ideal conditions for the growth and spread of fungal organisms. Like warts, nail fungus is almost impossible to eradicate without the cooperation of every member of a household. Children bring funguses home from camps and school locker rooms. Mom may get rid of her unsightly fungus, only to reinfect herself by stepping on Dad's towel. Treating nail fungus is very much like treating sexually transmitted diseases: It's useless to eradicate the infection in one person if someone else is going to ping-pong the bug right back to you.

Some nail funguses are accompanied by itching and pain, while others are simply a cosmetic problem, causing the nails to thicken and change color. Women generally want to treat cosmetic cases of nail fungus aggressively, while men tend to leave their nails alone if an unsightly appearance is the only symptom.

But appearance is *not* a negligible consideration: Advanced fungus nails are truly repellent, and many women are reluctant to participate in activities like swimming unless they can improve the appearance of their nails.

I see many, many more patients with nail fungus than I did when I began practicing, and I suspect that the increase is due to the proliferation of health clubs, school athletic programs, and nail parlors. All of these environments offer less-than-perfect (to put it mildly) sanitary conditions. The many advertisements on television for systemic oral antifungal medication attest to the size of the consumer market for nail fungus treatments. The newest drugs are highly effective, with far fewer side effects than the earlier generation. But they do affect the entire system and must therefore be taken under careful medical supervision. Ask your doctor about new, more effective *topical* antifungal solutions now becoming available.

SYMPTOMS

- Yellowing of the nail.
- Conspicuous thickening.
- Parts of the nail seem to be crumbling on the surface.
- The nail may jut away from its bed instead of lying in its usual flat position.
- A portion of the nail may break off, leading to inflammation or infection of the nail bed.
- In advanced cases, the nail may turn dark green in color.

FROM MY FILES

Sam and Gabriela, who have been married for fifteen years, offered a comical, and typical, example of the differing attitudes of women and men toward nail fungus. Sam had had an advanced case of nail fungus, involving several toes on both feet, for years. His feet didn't hurt or itch, and he watched with equanimity as his dark greenish nails thickened, cracked, crumbled, sloughed off, and were replaced by even more horny-looking sheaths.

Gabriela had managed for some years to avoid becoming infected, but that changed when they moved into a smaller apartment, where they shared a bathroom for the first time in their married life. She had only one fungus nail, but that was enough to bring her into the doctor's office, dragging Sam along in her wake. "I just avoided looking at his feet," she said, "but now that he's given this to me, I want the fungus out of our lives."

Since they had to share a bathroom, I dispensed my standard advice: Wash the floor and the tub with Clorox after every use and don't share towels or a bath mat. In treating such cases, I always begin with local rather than systemic medication. When patients come in with nail fungus, I tell them not to expect results overnight. Gabriela, however, was an exception, probably because she had only one fungus nail and came in almost as soon as she noticed it. I gently debrided her nail (pared down the thickened top layer) and prescribed a topical antifungal medication, which I recommended she use every night. Within just a few weeks, her nail looked perfectly normal—though it often takes two to three months to get results. However, I recommended that Gabriela continue to apply the medication for several months. One of the biggest mistakes patients make is to stop using topical antifungal ointments as soon as the symptoms improve. You must use the medication every day, for as many weeks or months as your podiatrist directs.

Sam, however, was a much more stubborn case. He had visible fungus on all of his nails and, although he had no pain and only mild itching around the cuticles, he had been walking around with the fungus for years. I told him he was unlikely to get rid of the fungus without systemic oral medication.

Systemic medications, as I've noted, must be taken under medical supervision. The two most commonly prescribed drugs (Sporanox and Lamisil) are contraindicated for people with any history of liver disease. And there can be negative drug interactions with certain antihistamines, anticoagulants, and steroids. Before prescribing these drugs, your podiatrist must take a careful medical history. Don't expect your doctor to prescribe such medications casually over the phone because you've heard about the benefits from a television ad.

Sam, however, was a good candidate for systemic antifungal medication. He had no history of liver disease, and he wasn't taking any other prescription drugs. And although he had agreed to treatment only because his wife insisted, it turned out that he was more bothered about the appearance of his nails than he had been willing to admit during his first visit. In fact, he told me, he was so ashamed of the way his feet looked that he always made a point of wearing his sneakers on the beach and stripping them off only at the water's edge. Furthermore, Sam and Gabriela had a twelve-year-old daughter, and he didn't want to pass on his nail fungus to her.

In cases like Sam's, the podiatrist must continue to debride the nails, and the patient must use topical medication, while taking the systemic drugs. It's not a quick or easy regimen, but within three months, Sam had normal-looking nails for the first time in a decade.

In the medical literature on nail fungus, many accounts stress the difficulty and uncertain success rate of treatment. I've had a great deal of success with both local and systemic medication, and I think that's because most of my patients are highly motivated and understand the importance of self-care to prevent recurrences. Expect to take oral medication for about two months. One thing is certain: You *will* contract nail fungus again unless you change the habits that exposed you to the infection the first time around.

PREVENTION AND SELF-CARE

Nail fungus is spread in the same fashion, and requires the same sanitary precautions, as athlete's foot.

■ Never walk around barefoot in a locker room or any other damp environment in which you don't know whose germs you're sharing. If you share a bathroom with someone who already has nail fungus, always wear shower clogs.

■ Don't wear the same socks home from the gym that you wore to work out. Damp socks are the perfect medium to transport fungal organisms from your health club to your home.

■ Don't wear athletic shoes all day. The synthetic materials used in most such shoes, unlike leather, don't allow your feet to breathe. Expose your feet to sunlight and air as much as possible.

But be aware that nail fungus is even harder to get rid of than athlete's foot, because the area under the nail is such a perfect incubator for infectious organisms. I strongly advise anyone who's already had fungus nails to shun commercial pedicures altogether. Learn how to give yourself sanitary pedicures at home (see Chapter 21, "The Beautiful Foot") and you won't have to risk exposure to another infection. Some of my patients tell me I'm a fanatic on this subject, but I've treated too many women who've gotten rid of their nail fungus after a long course of drug treatment only to turn up with a new infection after a pedicure.

14

Sprained Ankles and Shin Splints

WHAT GOES WRONG?

Along with Achilles tendinitis, sprained ankles and shin splints are the most common injuries that can be traced directly to exercise and sports. Sometimes (if you're unlucky), all three problems go together. The swollen ankle that so often accompanies Achilles tendinitis is really just a nonmedical term for a mild sprain.

SPRAINED ANKLES

Ankle sprains, like Achilles tendon injuries, come in varying degrees of severity. Most people—including athletes as well as women who sprain their ankles by stepping off a curb in high heels—hurt themselves by twisting the ankle inward. This process, responsible for nine out of ten sprains, involves a partial tear in the ligaments on the outside of the ankle.

If your ankle twists outward, the ligaments on the inside of the ankle may tear. This kind of sprain is much less common, and takes much longer to heal, than the typical sprain affecting your outside ankle ligaments. In an even smaller number of cases, there are ligament tears on both sides of the ankle.

A grade-three sprain is extremely severe and is often the result of a fall. It occurs most frequently in people who already have loose ligaments. That's one reason why pregnant women, whose ligaments are already laxer than usual as a result of hormonal changes, must take particular care to wear footwear that helps stabilize their ankles.

The main symptoms of a sprained ankle are swelling and pain. If you've done something to twist your ankle and you know it, you feel pain right away, followed by swelling. But not every sprain declares itself instantly; if you've recently increased your exercise level, your ankle may swell up and start to feel more tender over a period of days or weeks. This kind of sprain sneaks up on you; until the swelling is big enough and the ligaments torn enough to make you howl with pain, you probably won't be sure of what's happening. These "progressive" sprains might have been avoided by ice and rest at the first sign of swelling.

If you have swelling and pain in your ankle, seek medical attention immediately. X rays are necessary to rule out broken bones or joint dislocations, and your podiatrist will sometimes order an MRI to determine the extent of the ligament tear. It's important to evaluate the severity of the sprain as soon as possible because the degree of tearing determines how long you'll have to cut down on weight-bearing activity. Even after the most mild sprain, it may be six weeks before you can fully resume your weight-bearing exercise routine. Insufficient rest during a too-short rehab period can lead to a vicious cycle of recurrent sprains and the development of degenerative arthritis in your ankle joint.

SHIN SPLINTS

I can tell you from personal experience that shin splints really hurt—so much so that when the intense pain shoots through your lower legs for the first time, you may feel as if someone has hit you with a lead pipe. Here's why: Two important muscles are attached to the shin bone in your lower leg, and they literally tear away from the bone when you come up lame with shin splints. The greater the tear, the greater the pain. The tissue around the bone also becomes inflamed and swells.

I developed shin splints, as many people do, when I decided to turn myself overnight from a largely sedentary, overweight podiatrist and mother into a lean-and-mean jogger. My Achilles tendons were too tight for my new and overly ambitious exercise program; my feet, unaccustomed to the demands I was making on them, overpronated wildly and pitched my weight forward, and the muscles around the shin bone were badly overworked. Voilà! Within two weeks, my lower legs were swollen, and I couldn't even walk from my apartment to my office without pain. This was the end of my career as a runner and eventually led to my adopting a vigorous walking program (after my shin splints calmed down), better suited to my fitness goals and the state of my body.

Most of my patients develop shin splints exactly the way I did—by launching themselves into a demanding exercise program without adequate conditioning. However, even veteran exercisers can turn up with shin splints. If this happens to you, take a close look at your regular routine. Have you recently increased the difficulty of your workout? There's another possibility: Even if you're in excellent shape, shin splints may mean that you're not making allowances for the impact of aging on your body. The exercise routine that served you well at thirty-five may be too much for your body at forty-five.

SELF-CARE AND PREVENTION

For ankle sprains, assuming you've been X-rayed and a fracture has been ruled out, the outcome of medical treatment depends mainly on you—on your patience and your compliance with whatever physical therapy regimen is prescribed.

■ One of the first things to remember about ankle sprains is that they're treated with ice, not heat. For the first twelve hours after the injury (don't wait to see a doctor), elevate the ankle and apply an ice pack to the area for fifteen minutes out of every hour. *It's very important to keep the ice coming every hour during that first day.* Many people know enough to ice a sprain, but they're too impatient to keep up the self-treatment. Ice controls swelling by reducing the blood flow to the injured area. (Heat increases blood flow, exactly what you don't want in the immediate aftermath of an injury.)

It's also important that you not leave the ice on for more than twenty minutes at a time, because after that point, the blood vessels start to dilate in an effort to expand circulation. Use a kitchen timer to remind yourself when to stop icing. Flexible cold compress packs sold in drugstores—which reach freezing temperature but don't harden and are easy to mold to your body—are ideal for icing. You can keep them in your freezer and reuse them.

■ Elevate your foot while you're icing. Because the foot and ankle are so far from your heart, blood tends to pool in the injured area. If possible (this is tough for most people), try to keep your foot elevated continuously for twenty-four to forty-eight hours after the injury. In any event, do the best you can.

■ Rest may include crutches or a light air cast, and either of these will be combined with a compression bandage (sometimes for weeks). The compression keeps your ankle stable while enabling you to move around with less pain.

After the acute swelling subsides, your physical therapy program may include everything from heel cord stretching exercises to electrical stimulation designed to control residual swelling. Depending on the severity of the sprain, you can expect to have some swelling and pain for anywhere from two weeks to three months. If strenuous weight-bearing exercise is part of your regular routine, you must follow the recommendations of your physical therapist about how soon, and how vigorously, to resume your former activities.

■ Ice and rest are also the self-treatments of choice for bouts of shin splints. Achilles tendon and calf muscle stretches (pages 262-265) are as good for shin splints (both as prevention and cure) as for sprained ankles. Using an elastic bandage on your lower leg may help absorb some of the shock if you're over-pronating. When I started wearing orthotics in my walking shoes, I stopped having shin splints. But if the shin splints don't go away with ice and stretches, you need to see your podiatrist to make sure that you don't have a stress fracture in your lower leg.

A SPECIAL TIP FOR WOMEN . . .

If you're in your late forties and you've suddenly developed shin splints, you should have an X ray followed by a bone density test. Like stress fractures in the heels, the shins can provide an early warning of bone loss that may foreshadow osteoporosis in later years.

15

Tendinitis: Your Achilles Heel

WHAT GOES WRONG?

Your Achilles tendon is one of the most important pieces of soft tissue in your body—and one of the most vulnerable to injury. This tendon, also called the heel cord, is actually an extension of two lower calf muscles. It attaches your heel bone to the muscles that give it mobility and also allow you to rise on your toes. If your heel cord is too tight, you're bound to feel the strain elsewhere in your foot—especially in the plantar fascia ligament, which contracts and expands with every step.

To understand what a tight Achilles tendon does to your foot, think about the cords used to raise and lower venetian blinds. If the cords are untangled and of even length, the blinds go up and down smoothly, but if one piece of cord is twisted into a knot, you have trouble making the blinds move at all and they wind up in a crooked position. Although the heel cord and plantar fascia ligament aren't the same length, they must cooperate, like the pulleys and cords of a blind, to create smooth motion.

If the tendon is too tight, the plantar fascia ligament and

other soft tissues of the foot must stretch farther to enable you to put one foot in front of the other. Your foot rolls too far to the inside, overpronating to compensate. Over time, you're likely to feel pain and strain in the sole of the foot as well as the tendon and heel.

Achilles tendinitis is, quite simply, an inflammation that develops, either over time or suddenly, when your tendon isn't flexible enough to accommodate the pressure you're placing on your lower leg, ankle, and foot. Nature provides us with some latitude for slippage (and overstretching) in all of our tendons and joints: The popping when you crack your knuckles, which doesn't hurt but is an indication that you've made an extra demand on that part of your body, is a good example of the extra capacity for stretching.

Unfortunately, that stretch capacity—or leeway for error—diminishes as we age. When we overstretch a tendon at forty, it doesn't snap back the way it did when we were twenty. That's why people over forty are especially likely to strain their Achilles tendons if they begin an all-out fitness program suddenly rather than gradually. Overexercising isn't the only culprit: Many women hurt the tendon when they suddenly shift to flat shoes after a lifetime of wearing high heels. The tendon isn't used to stretching all the way to the ground, and it protests! As far as your foot is concerned, an unaccustomed stretch can be the equivalent of running an extra 10K.

SYMPTOMS

There are three basic degrees of severity in Achilles tendon injuries.

■ In a first-degree case—the least serious—you feel soreness at the back of (and often on either side of) your ankle. Sometimes there is a sharp pain in your calf, and you find it difficult to rise on your toes or put weight on your heels. You may also hear a clicking sound when you move your ankle, because there could be some damage to the soft tissue sheath that allows the tendon to glide smoothly over the bone. *Pay attention to these symptoms and get off your feet immediately, elevating and icing the area.* The worst mistake people make is to carry on with their usual routine, telling themselves that the pain will go away if they ignore it. If you do this, your strained ligament may tear.

■ Second-degree cases involve a partial tearing away of the tendon from the bone. These feel like a first-degree injury, only more so. If your pain lasts for more than two days, you must see a doctor for a diagnosis. (Experienced podiatric and orthopedic surgeons can often tell if you have a partial tear by feeling your ankle, but your doctor will probably recommend an MRI to make a definite diagnosis.) Second-degree injuries require a much longer period of immobility than first-degree cases. With a first-degree injury, you'll be able to walk (with the ankle tightly strapped) with little pain after forty-eight hours. A second-degree injury can take up to eight weeks to heal, and you may have to wear a flexible cast for several of those weeks.

■ In a third-degree injury, the tendon is completely torn away from the bone, and some of the adjacent muscles may also be ruptured. Only surgery can correct a complete rupture. If you have an Achilles tendon rupture, you will probably be referred to either a podiatric or an orthopedic surgeon. Make sure that your surgeon has extensive experience and specialized training in ankle-repair operations. (For further information on finding the right doctor, see Chapter 29, "How to Find the Best Medical Care for Your Lifestyle.")

Most Achilles tendon injuries don't fall into the third-degree category, and good orthopedists generally try noninvasive medical treatment before recommending an operation.

Note: A sprained ankle may accompany all types of Achilles tendon injuries.

FROM MY FILES

David, a first-time father at fifty, was running after a ball thrown by his three-year-old son when he felt a sharp pain at the back of his ankle. By the end of the day, the ankle had swollen up and David couldn't bear to put any weight on it. On Monday morning, he was in my office, wondering aloud how he could have done this to himself when he hadn't run very hard or very far.

This (fortunately) was a typical case of first-degree tendinitis. David had been smart enough to ice his ankle on and off all day Sunday, and the swelling had gone down somewhat by the time I saw him. But he was extremely unhappy when I told him that if he wanted to recover fully, and avoid reinjuring the tendon, he wouldn't be able to run or to carry his thirty-pound son on his shoulders for six to eight weeks. It's hard for people of any age to hear that they've hurt themselves because they're not in good enough shape to be doing the things they most want to do. In my experience, men have more trouble facing their physical limitations than women. In David's case, his reaction was intensified by his understandable desire to do everything younger fathers do with their children.

I told David that his need to rehabilitate the ankle provided an ideal opportunity for him to get in shape for years of activity with his son. After strapping the ankle tightly, I advised him to continue icing several times a day and to stay off the foot as much as possible for a week. I also inserted a heel lift inside his shoe to give the Achilles tendon a rest from its usual stretch.

When a woman who normally wears flat shoes turns up with Achilles tendinitis, I have her switch to one-inch heels. But it can be harder to treat women who normally wear extremely high heels: While they need lower-heeled shoes for stability during the healing period, their tendons may not be able to manage the extra stretch. It is, literally, a balancing act to settle on the right shoes for these patients.

For all patients, it's important to begin physical therapy as soon as possible. This may include electrical stimulation, ultrasound, and stretching exercises under the supervision of a therapist. People with injured Achilles tendons need to start their rehab under professional supervision so that they don't reinjure themselves by doing too much too soon. Eventually, the therapist will recommend a full at-home regimen of strengthening and stretching exercises for the hamstrings, lower calf muscles, and heel cord.

Even with a first-degree injury, you won't be able to engage in strenuous exercise for four to six weeks, depending on your general physical condition and the amount of effort you put into therapy. With second-degree injuries, the tendon itself doesn't heal for six to eight weeks, and you need another month of stretching exercises before you can return to your previous activity level.

In some instances, you'll be strongly advised against returning to your former regimen even after the injury is healed. If, for instance, you tore your Achilles tendon while you were running ten miles a day, it will take much longer than three months before you can hope to run the same distance without reinjuring yourself. And your therapist may tell you that it's much smarter to limit your run to five miles, regardless of how much time has passed and how good you feel.

I often have trouble convincing driven type A exercisers to take it easy (or easier). But that wasn't the case with David, who was interested in being an active father, not in proving that he had the body of a thirty-year-old. He was slightly overweight, and he dropped ten pounds during his rehab period, an immense asset to anyone trying to recover from any foot injury.

Most first- and second-degree injuries respond over time to this type of conservative medical treatment. But some patients (especially those with second-degree injuries) continue to have some pain for weeks—and pain relief is one of the most controversial subjects in podiatric and orthopedic practices.

Sometimes, especially if there is unusual swelling around the sheath of the Achilles tendon, your medical practitioner will recommend an anti-inflammatory steroid injection in the area. In many cases, this brings down the swelling and provides some immediate pain relief. But—and this is, in my view, an enormous "but"—a steroid injection may fool you into thinking the tendon is healing, and encourage reinjury, by masking the important warning signal provided by pain.

The widespread practice of treating injured athletes with steroids so that they can continue to play often leads to disastrous injuries: If your Achilles tendon (or any other tendon) hurts so much that you can't bear to put weight on it without repeated steroid injections, *you shouldn't be putting weight on it at all.* Many patients with painful Achilles tendon injuries ask for injections because they want to be back on their feet for a particular event. There's no doubt that a steroid shot might enable you to dance at a wedding or play ball during the company picnic—but at what cost? That dance on your injured tendon can translate into another three months in recovery. If your podiatrist or orthopedist refuses to give you an injection, please don't go looking for another practitioner who's more willing to say yes. Listen to what your doctor has to say about the danger of masking pain.

Over-the-counter anti-inflammatories containing aspirin or ibuprofen are usually adequate when pain recurs during the recovery period. I also prescribe stronger, nonsteroidal oral anti-inflammatories for patients whose injuries are healing normally but who have low pain tolerance. Expect some setbacks during your rehab period (especially if your tendon was partially torn). I recommend working with a professional physical therapist for some weeks. He or she will be able to tell whether your aches are caused by a renewed injury or whether they're simply part of the normal process of recovery.

PREVENTION AND SELF-CARE

■ Nearly all Achilles tendon injuries are preventable, and stretching exercises are the key. The exercises I recommend for plantar fasciitis are particularly helpful. If you can make time for only one set of warm-up exercises, these are the ones to choose.

Stretching and strengthening exercises for your hamstrings, large thigh muscles, and calf muscles are also important. Your ability to do such exercises varies greatly according to your physical condition, and you must consult a physical therapist before beginning a rehabilitative routine. Even if you're a veteran exerciser, you can benefit from professional advice during your rehabilitation period.

■ If you've had mild problems with either plantar fasciitis or Achilles tendinitis, a custom-made orthotic during exercise may prevent more strains by providing better support for your arch. One caution: The time to start using an orthotic is not right after you've been injured but when you're well on the way to recovery. Your podiatrist will explain how to "break in" your new orthotic devices.

■ Treat your foot and ankle with rest, ice, and elevation if you suspect you've injured your Achilles tendon and can't get to a doctor right away.

■ If you hurt your Achilles tendon in the course of an everyday act—say, stepping off a curb—you're probably wearing the wrong shoes. Men rarely suffer this kind of "everyday" injury, but women frequently twist their ankles in high, narrow heels that throw them off balance.

■ For both women and men, the majority of Achilles tendon injuries occur in the course of vigorous exercise. I can't stress enough the need to develop a sense of what's normal for *your* body—the difference between a slight strain due to overexertion and a real injury. Here are some questions to ask yourself if you've already sustained an injury.

—Has there been any recent change in my exercise routine? The answer to this isn't always obvious, because many people intensify their exercise level without realizing what they're doing. David, for example, hadn't thought about how much more time he was spending running and jumping as his son grew from a shaky two-year-old toddler into a highly coordinated—and unbelievably fast-moving—three-year-old.

—Am I adding specific motions that I wasn't doing before the injury? One of my female patients had taken tap-dancing classes for years and developed tendinitis when she switched to modern dance. The reason? Tap shoes have chunky heels, while modern dancers go barefoot or wear soft, completely flat slippers. Her Achilles tendon was too tight to accommodate the extra stretch.

—Are my athletic shoes in good condition?

■ Don't put off seeking medical help because you hope the pain will disappear by itself. It's particularly important to obtain an accurate diagnosis for soft-tissue injuries, because walking around on them can expand a minor tear into a major one.

The degree of pain doesn't always correlate with the seriousness of an injury. If the surrounding muscles are strong and you're in excellent overall physical condition, you may have minimal pain and still be able to walk around on an injury that would send someone else screaming to the emergency room. By contrast, acute pain doesn't necessarily mean that you've suffered the worst kind of tear: The injury may be exceptionally close to a nerve, or you may simply have a low tolerance for pain. If you can't put weight on your foot after two days, get medical help. Also, sometimes a stress fracture of the heel goes along with your Achilles tendinitis and sore ankle. In that case, your doctor will want to put you in a soft shoe cast while the tendon and the fracture heal.

A SPECIAL TIP FOR WOMEN . . .

Don't wear backless sandals or mules for extended walking, even if they feel comfortable on your feet. They destabilize your ankle, and that can lead to both sprains and Achilles tendinitis. Ordinary walking *is* exercise—whether you think of it that way or not—and you need support around your heel. Also, backless shoes subject the front of your foot to extra strain because you're using the muscles in your toes, consciously or unconsciously, to keep the shoes from falling off.

16

Warts

WHAT GOES WRONG?

Warts are benign tumors, caused by the human papilloma virus (HPV), that can appear on any skin surface or mucous membrane. These spongy lesions, of varying shapes and thicknesses, often itch violently, and when they emerge on areas subject to repeated friction and pressure—like the soles of the feet—they can become extremely painful. These growths on the soles are called plantar warts.

The HPV virus itself is highly contagious, especially in settings where people share towels or moist surfaces. The bathroom is a perfect setting for members of a household to spread their warts around: If one member of your family has recently developed a wart, you have to take strict sanitary precautions to avoid contamination. Children seem particularly vulnerable to HPV—either because they have lower resistance to the virus than adults or because hygiene isn't a top priority for most kids. If your child writes from camp and tells you his bunkmate has developed a "gross" wart, don't be surprised if your own darling brings a wart home as a souvenir of the summer.

Some warts disappear as mysteriously as they appear, without any effort on your part or intervention by a doctor. Others don't go away but don't grow either. Still others spread to adjacent areas, itching violently, and becoming infected if you scratch them (which it's hard not to do).

Why some people develop warts and others don't—even when they've clearly been exposed to the virus—is a mystery. I've been treating treating patients' warts for years without ever developing one on my fingers (yes, you can get warts on your hands from touching the warts on your feet). Yet I've had assistants who developed warts on their hands, even though they followed the same strict sanitary precautions that I always take. It's obvious to me that people are as variable in their susceptibility to HPV as they are to the ubiquitous viruses responsible for the common cold.

SYMPTOMS

- Itching. This is the main symptom associated with warts, but that doesn't tell you much because itching is also symptomatic of dozens of other dermatological conditions. Many people don't realize they have a wart because it's concealed by a larger, harder callus or corn. I often see these patients for the first time after they've infected a wart by scratching it.

- Your plantar wart won't necessarily hurt if it's not infected and you're wearing comfortable, padded shoes, but you will feel pain when you squeeze the lesion. If you squeeze an ordinary corn or callus, you're unlikely to feel anything at all.

- If you (unwisely) tried to get rid of the wart by paring it down with a sharp instrument at home, the growth probably bled. Warts can bleed quite profusely if they're traumatized, because of the presence of capillaries (the body's tiniest blood vessels) that are trapped by the tumor.

■ If your wart isn't covered by a callus, it probably comes in one of three varieties. First, there's the lone wart, which can range from a tiny dot to a larger growth of one-half to one and a half inches in diameter. The second common type of plantar growth is the mother-daughter formation, with one large wart and several smaller warts nearby. Sometimes the daughters encircle the mother wart. Finally, there's the mosaic wart, a large group of warts grouped together over the heel or ball of the foot.

Warts may change color, especially if they disappear spontaneously. In the process of receding, warts often become red and swell up—or, by contrast, they turn black and harden. Many people, remembering that "any change in a wart or mole" is listed among the signs of skin cancer, understandably become alarmed by these shifts in coloration. While cancerous tumors on the foot are extremely rare—and in fact, I've never seen one masked as a wart—you should see a podiatrist or a dermatologist if your wart hasn't been medically diagnosed. A definite diagnosis will set your mind at rest, and you'll be guarding against the tiny chance that your growth is something other than an ordinary wart.

FROM MY FILES

When eleven-year-old Jenny D'Angelo (not her real name) came home from camp with large warts on her heels, her mother did what most people do: She tried to get rid of the unsightly growths with over-the-counter medication. Sometimes these nonprescription preparations work, but they didn't do anything for Jenny—and Mrs. D'Angelo soon developed a wart on her finger. (She probably touched her daughter's wart when it was in a "spreading" phase while applying the medication.) Within two months, both Mrs. D'Angelo and her husband had developed plantar warts on their feet. Clearly, the family members were passing warts back and forth to one another, probably by walking around on the same damp bathroom floors.

The first step toward ridding the family of warts was a rigid cleanup routine (there's no getting around this). I told the D'Angelos that each family member must scrub down the bathroom with household bleach after every use. And no walking around barefoot, just in case a stray viral cell might be lurking, waiting to work its way inside a heel fissure. (Some doctors consider this routine excessive, but I've found that it's almost impossible for a couple or a family to get rid of warts without following these sanitary measures. Furthermore, I've had patients who were "wart-free" for more than a year and who admitted sheepishly, when they turned up back in my office with a new crop, that they'd started skipping the bleach.

HPV, like so many viruses, can't be knocked out of your system by a prescription drug. (Medical history has demonstrated that viruses—smallpox and polio are the prime examples—can be eradicated only by a vaccine that creates immunity.) What we can do is remove the warts locally and reduce the possibility of recurrence through sanitary precautions.

Because nonprescription compounds hadn't worked for the D'Angelos, we decided on cryotherapy treatments as the best way to get rid of the growths. In cryotherapy, the podiatrist freezes the wart with liquid nitrogen and carefully debrides it (shaves it down with a sterile instrument). This is an absolutely painless (the freezing process numbs you) office procedure.

It will probably take several sessions to get rid of your warts (depending on the size and number), because the growths must be debrided in stages in order to avoid harming healthy tissue. Also, new warts may still crop up in the course of treatment because the wart was already in a "spreading" stage—about to give birth to new warts—when you began cryotherapy.

The D'Angelos came in once a week for cryotherapy, and it took six weeks to banish all of their warts. While cryotherapeutically treated areas don't hurt afterward, they do need to be protected with sterile padding because the surface is much more vulnerable to infection during the treatment process.

Warts can also be removed with a laser, which kills the abnormal warty tissue by the heat from a beam of infrared light. This procedure can be performed only by a board-certified podiatric surgeon (not all podiatrists are authorized to perform surgery).

The wart is numbed with local anesthesia, and the laser beam is directed around the perimeter. Then the center is scooped out and any bleeding can be stopped with a sponge. Most patients are fully satisfied with the results of this procedure. However, it's impossible for even the most skilled surgeon to use a laser without destroying some healthy tissue along with the wart. It takes a few weeks for the area to heal fully. And there are some parts of the feet, like the sole, where it's inappropriate to employ the laser because the layer of skin and cushioning is so thin there. In most instances, cryotherapy works very well. I reserve the laser for intractable cases in which every other treatment has failed and the wart is painful (and often a significant source of embarrassment).

It's been a year since the D'Angelos completed their cryotherapy, and no one has had a recurrence. Mrs. D'Angelo sent Jenny back to camp this year with slippers and a large bottle of bleach.

PREVENTION AND SELF-CARE

■ If you know you have a plantar wart (you may not know what it is the first time, but if you've already had one, you'll recognize it when you see it again), clean up with bleach and use separate towels for your feet and the rest of your body. Even if you live alone, this is a good idea. Use a different color or size towel for your feet, so you don't get confused.

■ Commercial, over-the-counter pads and compounds in which the active ingredient is *salicylic acid*—a caustic solution that dissolves tissue of all kinds—are often useful. I recommend that you use preparations containing no more than 60 percent salicylic acid (ask your pharmacist if you're in doubt) because the acid dissolves healthy as well as dead tissue. You're much more likely to hurt yourself with products containing a higher concentration.

■ Both pads and liquids take about two weeks to work with repeated applications. You'll notice dead skin forming; shave it down lightly each time with a pumice stone or abrasive brush. Whatever you do, *don't touch the wart with your bare hands!*

■ There are stronger, more caustic commercial substances available—from preparations containing a higher concentration of salicylic acid to silver nitrate and sulfuric acid (yes, some people really do try to apply sulfuric acid to their own feet)—but I strongly suggest that you consult a podiatrist if your wart doesn't respond to standard products in two or three weeks.

■ Here's a home remedy of mine that some patients have found effective. Make a paste of four tablespoons bottled water (to ensure sterility), five aspirins, one vitamin E capsule, and one teaspoon of liquid vitamin A (available in any health food store or pharmacy). Apply this paste directly to the wart, put your foot in a plastic bag for fifteen minutes, and gently remove any dead skin with a pumice stone.

■ If your wart isn't painful or itchy, and its appearance doesn't bother you, you can just leave it alone. But I find that most people—men as well as women—are as concerned about the appearance as they are about any pain and scratchiness. As Jenny D'Angelo remarked, "I've only seen something that looked like this on the noses of witches in fairy-tale books."

A SPECIAL TIP FOR WOMEN . . .

Never allow a pedicurist in a nail parlor to use a pumice stone or any other instrument on your plantar warts. Some nail and beauty parlors even advertise wart removal as a specialty. (This may or may not be legal in your state.) In a nonsterile setting, the pedicurist may inadvertently add fungal organisms or bacteria to your viral warts. If she goes too far with a sharp instrument, the trapped capillaries may burst and bleed heavily.

17

If You Need an Operation: What's New in Diagnosis and Surgery

While I've emphasized my preference for conservative, non-surgical treatment of most foot pain, there are times when an operation is the only real remedy. I find that for many of my patients, especially those under fifty, foot surgery is their first encounter with the new world of high-tech medicine. Whether you have a painful bunion or a ruptured Achilles tendon, it's important for you to become a better-educated medical consumer so you can ask the right questions, understand your surgeon's answers, and make an informed decision.

Twenty years ago, when I was a surgical resident, patients undergoing even the most routine foot operations were hospitalized for at least one night. If you were having a bunion removed (then, as now, one of the most common foot surgeries), you received general anesthesia and woke up with a hard plaster cast at the end of your leg. For six weeks, your foot was immobilized. When the cast was removed, your foot hurt, because your muscles already had begun to atrophy as a result of the prolonged immobilization. Three months passed before you could walk without some degree of pain, and it took at least another nine months of physical therapy for you to resume vigorous exercise. Unless you happened to be a magnificent young physical specimen with extraordinary recuperative powers, there was no way around this long and arduous recovery period. Small wonder that many people preferred the pain of a badly inflamed bunion to the pain of surgery and its aftermath!

Today, unless the case is especially complicated or there's another medical condition warranting overnight hospitalization, I remove bunions in my office. (Even if the operation is performed in a hospital, most patients go home the same day after spending a few hours in a special ambulatory recovery room.) When a patient has had local or IV anesthesia in my office, she's usually alert enough to leave an hour or so after the surgery, accompanied by a relative or friend.

Three days later, the recovering patient is walking around in a soft surgical boot. The first week after surgery, I put most of my patients on a special reclining bicycle that enables them to lie back and exercise the calf, ankle, and foot muscles without putting any pressure on the healing area. Most healthy adults are back in normal shoes, and able to walk at an ordinary pace without pain, in about six weeks.

The transformation of foot surgery during the past two decades has been achieved as a result of improvements in anesthesia, diagnostic techniques, and surgical instruments themselves. The MRI (magnetic resonance imaging), which provides a computer-generated portrait revealing the extent and precise location of soft-tissue injuries, has become widely available as a diagnostic tool only during the past decade. Before MRIs, a doctor could only guess about the severity of a soft tissue tear—and about whether it was likely to heal without surgery.

The improvement in surgical instruments is just as marked as the change in diagnostic tools. During my training period, we had to make a large incision in order to see what we were doing inside the foot—and we were wielding the surgical equivalent of chisels and hammers. We did, in fact, employ a small hammer to fracture the bones that needed to be realigned during bunion surgery. Today, by contrast, we use delicate electrical reciprocating blades to create a fracture so precise that it's barely visible on a postsurgical X ray after the bone is healed.

Computerized videocameras project microscopic images to guide the surgeon: In other words, we no longer have to cut your foot wide open to see what's going on inside. These procedures are the podiatric equivalents of laparoscopic abdominal operations, which allow surgeons to remove benign ovarian cysts, gallstones, and even appendixes without making a large abdominal incision. The laparoscope, which enables the surgeon to view various areas of the abdominal cavity, serves the same purpose as the computer-assisted endoscope in plantar fasciotomies and the arthroscope in ankle and knee surgeries.

There's much less bleeding and much less destruction of soft tissue, which not only minimizes postsurgical pain but also shortens the healing process. On an average, my surgical patients today heal in about half the time it would have taken them to recover from the same operation twenty years ago.

Here are some of the most common tests and surgical procedures your doctor may suggest.

MRI (MAGNETIC RESONANCE IMAGING)

An MRI maps the soft tissues of your body by transforming low-energy radiowaves, through the use of a complex magnet, into a computer-generated image. The MRI can identify the precise location of problems in ligaments, tendons, and blood vessels. It may also sometimes reveal microscopic hairline fractures that have been missed by conventional X rays. MRI tests are painless but not pleasant (especially for claustrophobics), since they involve inserting part or all of your body into a machine that resembles a tight tunnel. The loud *thump-thump* of the machine while it's in operation led one of my patients to remark that the test was his idea of being buried alive on a construction site.

An MRI can take anywhere from twenty minutes to two hours, depending on how many views of the particular body part are required. Although the MRI is no one's idea of fun, it's essential for proper diagnosis of many kinds of serious injuries. In many instances, this procedure helps you and your doctor decide *against* surgery. For example, the size of an Achilles tendon tear revealed on an MRI provides a good indicator of your chances of healing smoothly without an operation. And if you do need to have the tendon surgically repaired, the MRI is the equivalent of a map. Operating on soft tissue before MRIs was the equivalent of flying without instruments.

ULTRASOUND

Ultrasound machines of various kinds are used both in diagnosis and treatment. In an MRI, radiowaves are transformed into an image with the aid of computers; ultrasound devices use sound waves to do the same thing. If you're pregnant, you'll probably see your baby *in utero* for the first time via ultrasound. Podiatrists use ultrasound (often before surgery) to determine whether there's normal blood flow to the foot.

Ultrasound is most familiar to postsurgical rehab patients not as a diagnostic tool but as a way of improving circulation in the foot through deep heating. It's also used in a procedure called phonophoresis, in which the sound waves are used to infuse anti-inflammatory medication into an injured area without an injection. Phonophoresis is especially helpful in the treatment of children and adults who are particularly fearful of injections.

NERVE CONDUCTION VELOCITY STUDIES

Nerve conduction tests, which are painless, involve placing electrodes on the skin to determine whether various parts of your foot are receiving nerve signals in a normal pattern. Your podiatrist is likely to do a nerve conduction analysis if numbness—which could indicate some impairment of the neurological or vascular systems—is one of your symptoms. If your nerve conduction velocity tests are abnormal but you've never been diagnosed with a systemic disease that would explain the results, you may be referred to a neurologist or vascular specialist.

EMG (ELECTROMYOGRAM)

This test is performed in a special facility, and it is mildly uncomfortable. Needles are inserted in the muscle (though it doesn't hurt after the insertion), and your muscular strength is tested by analyzing contractions. I don't order this test often, but it is necessary if there are signs that you might have a systemic neuromuscular disease.

ENDOSCOPIC SURGERY

The endoscope is an instrument that enables a surgeon to directly visualize the inside of the foot on a video screen while she's operating through a small incision. The plantar fasciotomy, in which the plantar fascia ligament is released to relieve the pain associated with heel spurs, is perhaps the best example of what the endoscope can do. In classical heel spur surgery in the past, a large, long incision was necessary to remove the bone spur and sever the ligament. Now the spur is left alone, and the ligament is released through an incision of just an inch or so.

ARTHROSCOPIC SURGERY

Arthroscopy is now the surgical method of choice for a large proportion of operations involving the shoulder, elbow, knee, and ankle joints. The arthroscope is another of the new breed of computer-assisted instruments that allow a doctor to see into a joint and operate through an extremely small incision. If you have torn cartilage in your ankle, it will most likely be repaired through an arthroscopic procedure. Arthroscopic operations are also performed to repair many Achilles tendon tears. However, there are major reconstructive surgeries, usually necessitated by severe injuries, that can be conducted only in the traditional fashion through a large open incision.

QUESTIONS YOU SHOULD ASK YOUR DOCTOR BEFORE FOOT SURGERY

Is there any downside to delaying surgery while trying a more conservative treatment?

The answer depends entirely on the location and nature of the injury. Some injuries almost certainly get better with con-

What You Should Know About Anesthesia

The shift from general to local anesthesia for most foot operations has been a great boon. Patients who haven't been unconscious for hours are quicker to recover—not only from the immediate impact of the surgery but during the ensuing days and weeks. There are five basic kinds of nongeneral anesthesia used in foot surgery.

■ *Local injection or toe block* (much like the use of Novocaine for filling teeth), for surgeries that don't extend beyond the base of the toes. You can expect a toe block if you're having a minor procedure to clear up a nail infection.

■ *Ankle block* (of the posterior tibial nerve), numbs the entire foot. In many cases, I use an ankle block for bunionectomies.

■ *Epidural block* around the nerves of the lower back (most commonly used during childbirth). It's frequently used for ankle surgery and for major operations in the back of the foot, because an ankle block won't numb the area sufficiently.

■ *Spinal block*, in which anesthesia is injected into the spinal cord.

■ *IV sedation*, usually combining a painkiller and a muscle relaxant. You probably won't be aware of anything during the procedure, and you definitely won't feel any pain. Unlike old-fashioned general surgical anesthesia, the effects of IV sedation wear off quickly and enable you to go home soon after the procedure.

General anesthesia is now used primarily for major reconstructive surgeries that take many hours. There are also some systemic medical conditions—multiple sclerosis among them—that make general anesthesia safer than local injections. And if you have severe degenerative arthritis in your lower back, your doctor may recommend general anesthesia because an epidural or spinal block might well exacerbate your back pain.

servative nonsurgical treatment, while others get worse if they're not operated on as soon as possible. Somewhere in the middle are traumas (many soft-tissue tears fall into this category) that don't necessarily improve under conservative methods but don't get worse while you're waiting for the outcome. If rest, ice, physical therapy, and other nonsurgical intervention don't seem to be helping, your podiatrist will probably order some of the diagnostic tests I've described.

How long will I have to wear a cast, use crutches, etc., after the operation?

How much pain will I be in for the first forty-eight hours after the surgery?
Your surgeon won't be able to give a definitive answer to this question, since pain is highly individual and subjective, but she will be able to give you best- and worst-case scenarios.

When can I reasonably expect to walk unaided without pain?

If my work is physically demanding or I'm accustomed to engaging in active sports, how long should I allow before I can realistically expect to return to those activities?
You might also ask your doctor what expectations should be considered *unreasonable*.

How quickly is hospital backup available if something goes wrong?
Obviously, this question applies only if surgery is being performed in a doctor's office or freestanding ambulatory clinic.

How many operations of this particular type has the surgeon performed?

What percentage of patients have emerged with what the surgeon considers a "best-case" outcome?

This is an important question, because while no surgeon can guarantee that one patient will have exactly the same outcome as another, doctors do and should have a very clear idea of the *percentage* of their patients who obtain satisfactory results.

PART III

Your Feet and the Rest of Your Body

18

Arthritis and Your Feet

WHAT GOES WRONG?

Arthritis, a general term for inflammation of the joints, is involved in a significant number of painful foot problems in people over forty. There are actually more than 100 forms of arthritis—some extremely painful, some merely annoying. In an arthritic joint, the cartilage—soft tissue that serves as a buffer between bones—has thinned out. The tissue may dry, crack, and split, exposing bones and causing them to grind against one another. The crackling sound people sometimes hear when they flex an arthritic knee or ankle is the grinding of bone on bone.

Swelling occurs when the synovial cells, which line the joint, become enlarged and too much fluid accumulates in the tissue. These joints, swollen with excess fluid, can become hot and extremely painful to the touch. When you recall that your foot has thirty-five small joints, it should be easy for you to understand why systemic arthritis often attacks "feetfirst." The ankle, big toe, and metatarsal joints are particularly susceptible to arthritic flare-ups. There's nothing predictable about the course of this disease. Some people have occasional bouts of inflammation, while others experience pain every day. Some patients' joints degenerate steadily with age, while others hit a plateau and don't get much worse.

Osteoarthritis

Of the many forms of arthritis, age-related osteoarthritis is unquestionably the most common. More than 90 percent of people over sixty have some degree of arthritis, though the absence of arthritic changes in the lucky 10 percent has led to speculation about "fountain of youth" gene therapy in the future. For now, nearly all of us can expect to contend with arthritis as we grow older.

Trauma—whether the result of a single bad accident or cumulative wear and tear—can set off and exacerbate arthritis at any age. X rays of professional athletes in their early thirties often reveal arthritic changes that aren't usually seen until the sixties and seventies. And specialists have found that arthritis is even more of a problem for athletes in sports that impose greater physical demands than they did in the past.

As recently as fifteen years ago, for example, female Olympic figure skaters didn't do triple jumps. Now every world-class skater is expected to pack a program with triples (in which the skater takes off on one foot and rotates three full times in the air before landing on the other). This change has led to more traumatic injuries, and earlier arthritis, of the foot, ankle, knee, and hip of skaters' landing legs. Similarly, I often see early arthritic changes in the feet of patients who've been running since they were in their teens.

For women, high heels have now been shown to encourage osteoarthritis in knees because they prevent the ankles from working as they should to stabilize the knee joints. D. Casey Kerrigan, an assistant professor at Harvard Medical School who specializes in rehabilitation, used specialized laboratory equipment to analyze the forces generated in the knees of women who habitually wore high heels. She found that the rotational forces compressing the inner part of the knee joint were 23 percent higher when women walked in high heels than when they walked barefoot. Heels also increased the strain on the smaller joint between the kneecap and the underlying thigh bone, a frequent site of osteoarthritis in women.

One of the many mysteries about osteoarthritis is that there's no absolute correlation between the severity of degenerative joint changes and the degree of pain. I can look at X rays of two people with relatively similar arthritic changes in their toe joints, and one experiences only an occasional ache, easily relieved by over-the-counter anti-inflammatory medication, while the other feels frequent and acute pain in spite of taking much stronger prescription drugs.

Rheumatoid Arthritis

This is the second most common form of arthritis and may strike at any age. Specialists now believe that rheumatoid arthritis may be attributable to an immune deficiency or even a virus (or both). Although rheumatoid arthritis has many of the same symptoms as osteoarthritis, it is not caused by ordinary wear and tear. Women are three times as likely as men to suffer from the disease, so there may be a genetic factor. Although more than a third of people with rheumatoid arthritis have only one attack of pain and inflammation, half suffer through recurrent bouts. In the most severe cases, the degenerative process is so acute that muscle imbalance, joint dislocation, and circulatory impairment are common. Severe bunions, chronically swollen ankles, claw toes (a combination hammertoe and mallet toe, caused by a buckling of two joints) are just a few of the podiatric complications of chronic rheumatoid arthritis.

Gout

Gout is another extremely painful form of arthritis, attributable to an accumulation of uric acid crystals in the joints. Gout sufferers have been portrayed (and often ridiculed) in drawings—usually caricatures of fat men with swollen toes—since the Middle Ages. There seems to be both a hereditary and a hormonal susceptibility to gout. It's much more common in men than in women and rarely occurs in women before menopause, which probably means that estrogen protects against the disease. Gout symptoms seem to be aggravated by a diet rich in high-fat meats and alcohol—one reason why sufferers have often been mocked. Since only the rich could afford this diet in centuries past, gout was long considered a disease of the wealthy. King Henry VIII was probably the most famous royal gout victim.

Gout loves to attack the big toe, and the pain can be so acute that the sufferer can't even stand to have a sheet over his foot. Some recent studies have cast doubt on the traditional association between gout and a too-rich diet, but I don't believe them. I can't count the number of times I've seen young men (in their thirties and forties) with their first attack of gout, only to learn that they'd been to a party the night before and consumed large quantities of beef, red wine, and dessert. This can't be just coincidence!

Many first-time gout sufferers call a podiatrist rather than their internist, because they don't know what's happening and assume that they've injured their toe. I can usually diagnose gout myself because the concentration of uric acid crystals is easily visible under a microscope. You need to see a rheumatologist if you have gout, and the acute inflammation of the toe generally clears up after only a few days of systemic anti-inflammatory medication. The rheumatologists I know all believe there is an association between gout attacks and certain foods, and they'll discuss your diet with you.

. . .

Some of my arthritic patients are already being treated by a rheumatologist. Others, however, are seeking help from me for what they think is a routine, localized foot problem, and they're often extremely upset when I tell them that they may have arthritis. When I suspect that arthritis is the real culprit, I do a blood test to look for certain markers for arthritis. If they show up in the results, I refer the patient to a rheumatologist. I can help an arthritic patient handle the foot symptoms, but only a rheumatologist can provide proper treatment for the systemic disease that's causing the trouble.

FROM MY FILES

Rebecca, forty-five, has a severe case of rheumatoid arthritis and was referred to me by her internist. Although Rebecca had developed a great many foot problems as a result of her rheumatoid condition, she came to see me because she had begun to experience numbness alternating with shooting pain, especially at night. The pains were sharp enough to disturb her sleep.

I suspected a condition called tarsal tunnel syndrome (the podiatric equivalent of the better-known carpal tunnel syndrome, which causes pain and numbness in hands and is associated with repetitive stress injury). In tarsal tunnel syndrome, the ligament around the ankle tightens and constricts the passageway of the major (posterior tibial) nerve leading from the calf to the foot.

The back of Rebecca's ankle was visibly swollen, and she had soft-tissue scarring in many of her joints as a result of her rheumatoid condition. A nerve conduction velocity test, in which an electrode is placed on the skin, revealed that the "messages" from the posterior tibial nerve weren't being transmitted to the foot on a steady basis, which accounted for the alternating numbness and flashes of pain. I tried anti-inflammatory injections to reduce the swelling and physical therapy to increase circulation, but these didn't work. Finally, Rebecca and I (with the concurrence of her doctor) decided on surgery to free the trapped posterior tibial nerve. In this operation, performed under local anesthetic, the tight tissues are released through a small incision. At the same time, some of the excess scar tissue is cleaned out of the tarsal tunnel.

Until the postsurgical swelling subsides, numbness and pain may persist (though to a lesser degree) for several months. In Rebecca's case, the results were better than anticipated; both symptoms subsided within weeks rather than months. The key to this result, I believe, was Rebecca's quick response to new sensations in her foot. One obstacle to effective intervention in severe cases of arthritis affecting the foot (whether of the rheumatoid or the more common age-related variety) is that the patient, accustomed to joint pain, ignores a change in her condition.

Whatever kind of arthritis you have, it's most important that your general condition be controlled with appropriate medical treatment. Rebecca's was a somewhat unusual case. In most instances, I advise people with arthritic feet to employ the commonsense self-care methods I recommend for many painful foot conditions.

SELF-CARE AND PREVENTION

For most of us, there's no way to prevent some arthritic changes as we grow older. But there are ways to lessen the severity of the symptoms and accommodate ourselves to them in order to go on with an active life.

■ All types of arthritis, of whatever degree of severity, call for shoes with extra cushioning on the bottom. Remember, you're losing cartilage in your joints, and cartilage is the body's shock absorber. Well-padded shoes will not correct deformities produced by arthritic changes in your foot, but they will reduce the pressure on the area.

■ Since the toe joints are so often affected by arthritis, be particularly careful to buy shoes with a comfortably wide and deep toebox. And your shoes should have uppers made of soft materials—suede instead of polished leather, for instance—whenever possible.

■ Moist heat and soaking in hot water have been recommended since time immemorial for arthritic pain. They have a temporary, but deeply soothing, effect.

■ Gentle exercise is now recognized as an extremely important element in the management of all forms of arthritis. In Chapter 28, "The Well-Exercised Foot," I outline a program of small, easy exercises to help maintain flexibility in your feet. I strongly urge all of my patients with arthritis to consult a physical therapist or trainer for advice on an exercise program custom-tailored for joint problems. Many local institutions, including Ys across the country, offer special exercise classes for people with arthritis. The common thread in all of these programs is the need to maintain flexibility without imposing high-impact pressure on the joints.

■ If your joints frequently swell up after activity, allow time for icing afterward.

■ If you're taking anti-inflammatory medicine—over-the-counter or prescription—follow the dosage guidelines rigorously. Side effects from these drugs include ulcers and bleeding in the intestinal tract, and you're more likely to develop these problems if you exceed the normal dosage.

19

Diabetes and Your Feet

WHAT GOES WRONG?

Diabetes, a serious and incurable disorder in which the body is unable to metabolize sugar properly, meant an early death sentence before the discovery of insulin in the 1920s. Now, with regular insulin therapy and diet control, most diabetics can lead normal lives. Type 1 (juvenile) diabetes, which declares itself in childhood, is the most severe form of the disease and must usually be controlled with insulin injections. Type 2 (adult-onset diabetes) generally presents itself after age thirty and can often be controlled with diet and oral insulin. Both forms of the disease are serious and require constant vigilance. Meticulous podiatric care is vital to effective management of diabetes over a lifetime.

Whether you have type 1 or type 2 diabetes, you are at high risk for serious foot troubles; in fact, a seemingly minor foot infection may be one of the first symptoms of the disease. Most of my diabetic patients are referred to me by their medical doctors, but occasionally I spot a healthy-looking young adult who has no idea that the sore spot on her foot means there's something really wrong. I hate telling these patients what I suspect, but they're truly lucky to have received a warning signal before diabetes impairs their health in more serious ways.

The main reason for the prevalence of foot problems in diabetics is that the disease impairs circulation. Nerves and tissues, particularly in the body's extremities, don't get an adequate supply of blood. This can cause symptoms ranging from numbness to severe infection. Fourteen million Americans have diabetes, and studies have shown that diabetes-related foot problems are the *third leading cause of hospitalization* in the United States.

Peripheral neuropathy, which cuts down on the blood supply to your nerves, causes the muscles of the foot to atrophy and lose sensation. This can promote the development of infections and ulcers. Of course, this loss of sensation is dangerous because it makes diabetics ignore symptoms that would alarm people who have full sensation in their feet. Peripheral neuropathy can sometimes lead to a far more serious condition called Charcot arthropathy, in which the foot swells and multiple bones begin to crumble. If this condition is not diagnosed early and treated aggressively, it can lead to amputation.

SYMPTOMS

If you know you have diabetes, *any* minor swelling, discoloration, visible sore, or pain should mean an immediate visit to the podiatrist. Your doctor undoubtedly has emphasized the importance of prompt medical attention for foot problems. Don't ever say, "Oh, it's nothing," and let it go. With your compromised circulation, a tiny sore can swiftly turn into an oozing infection. It's impossible to catalog the array of foot symptoms that merit prompt attention in diabetics, but here is a partial list:

- Burning feet
- Cold feet
- Thickening or discoloration of a nail (similar to nail fungus)
- Numbness
- Fissures
- Any rash or itching
- Soreness around the nails
- Any injury to the foot

Do these symptoms sound too ordinary to merit attention? For nondiabetics, many of them are. If you sprain your ankle and you're a healthy adult, you might well try rest and an ice pack before you call a doctor. If you're a diabetic, you can't do that. Because your circulation is compromised, it takes more aggressive treatment to get the swelling down—and it's more important to bring the swelling down as soon as possible.

FROM MY FILES

Tony, a longtime patient in his early thirties, exemplifies what a diabetic can do to keep his feet and the rest of his body in top-notch shape for a life that's active by any standard. Tony has been an insulin-dependent diabetic since childhood—he now uses an insulin pump—but he has always participated in active sports. He continues to play tennis and softball, and I think his regular exercise routine is the main reason why his feet are in so much better shape than many of the diabetic feet I treat. Tony also keeps his weight down, something that's particularly important, as extra pounds cause even greater stress on diabetic joints that already have a compromised blood supply.

Nevertheless, the skin on Tony's feet is extremely dry, and he has a tendency to develop painful fissures in his heels—an indication that his circulation, while better than the average diabetic's, is still impaired. Tony comes in every five weeks for a meticulous examination to make sure that he hasn't missed any fissures or microscopic breaks in the skin. And he moisturizes his feet with a copper-based cream I mix myself. (In addition to having healthy skin, Tony has some of the most attractive-looking feet of any man I know!)

I expect to see more diabetics like Tony, people who cope with this disease so effectively that it hasn't stopped them from doing anything they want to do. The development of new ways to administer insulin, in patient-monitored doses, makes that more likely. But all diabetics need to be as utterly meticulous—some would say obsessive—as Tony is about his feet in order to avoid severe podiatric complications.

PREVENTION AND SELF-CARE

- Inspect your feet carefully, in a bright light, at least once a day for any change in texture or color. Be sure to check between your toes too.

- Don't ever walk around barefoot. Because the diabetic foot may suffer from some loss of sensation, you could step on something sharp without realizing it. Another reason not to go barefoot is that you should keep your feet extremely clean at all times.

- Don't wear shoes without stockings or socks.

- Don't smoke or drink caffeinated beverages. Nicotine and caffeine constrict your blood vessels.

- Don't ever use over-the-counter corn and callus removers. All minor foot problems must be treated in a sterile medical setting. And it should go without saying: No nail parlors for you.

- I recommend that you don't even trim your own toenails. If you're seeing a podiatrist regularly—which you should be—she can take care of that for you. If you're in a situation where you absolutely must cut your own nails, don't cut them shorter than the tips of the toes. And never trim your own cuticles.

■ Your doctor has probably already told you that exercise is important to maintain circulation. The foot flexibility exercises in Chapter 28, "The Well-Exercised Foot," help prepare you for a more vigorous routine worked out under the supervision of your doctor and a physical therapist.

20

Your Feet and Your Aching Back

WHAT GOES WRONG?

There's an intimate connection between lower back pain and foot pain. If you have chronic trouble with your back, it's almost impossible to escape foot problems: As you walk in an unnatural position to compensate for the pain in your back, you're bound to place uneven pressure on your feet. Corns, blisters, and aching arches are just a few of the foot problems that can be traced to your spine. The reverse is equally true. If you've been walking around for years on an inflamed bunion, you've been trying, consciously and unconsciously, to avoid the painful spot. The alignment of your knees, hips, and lower back can't help but be affected. Which came first, the chicken or the egg? In my view, it doesn't really matter. If you're being medically treated for back pain, you should also have a thorough podiatric examination. Many orthopedists suggest this to their back patients, but I've sometimes encountered patients who've been going to back doctors for years without ever having had their feet checked out.

Here's just a partial list of what can go wrong in the delicate connection between the back and the feet.

■ *You have unusually high arches.* People with very high arches place an unusual degree of pressure on their heels when they walk, sending shocks straight up to the base of the spine. (Their gait poses a direct contrast to that of people with fallen arches, who overpronate and shift too much weight to the balls of the feet.) Because your heel has been absorbing extra pressure throughout your life, it probably is deficient in fatty tissue padding by the time you enter your thirties. Over time, the dearth of shock absorbers in the high-arched foot is bound to affect the lower back.

■ *Flat feet.* Flat feet, or fallen arches, can also throw your back out of whack. When you overpronate and shift too much weight toward the balls of your feet, the muscles of your legs and back have to work harder to prevent you from shifting further out of balance. High heels are a major factor in this equation, because they concentrate your weight, already shifted too far forward, in an even smaller area of your forefoot.

And yes, if your high arches fall, you'll have the worst of both worlds. The cushioning on your heels will be worn down from years of walking on high arches, but you'll have entirely new problems as a result of your sagging arches and plantar fascia ligament.

■ *Bunions.* If bunions are in their early stages and don't hurt you, they're not likely to be a cause of back pain. But if your bunions have been hurting for years, the muscles of your back are likely to have been pushed out of alignment as you tried to ease the pain in your feet.

■ *Leg length discrepancy.* Many people are born with one leg slightly longer than the other. You may not be aware of any disparity—in most instances, it isn't visible—but over a lifetime, one hip will tilt slightly and your spine will curve as you attempt to even out your walking surface. The uneven pressure means pain for both your back and your feet.

■ *Arthritic changes.* Age-related arthritic changes in your feet, ankles, and knees can exacerbate arthritis in your lower back (and vice versa). Think of a flexible ladder, anchored firmly so that you can climb straight up and down with no trouble. Now think of just one of the rungs being wrenched out of place, so that you have to keep twisting and turning to complete the climb without falling off. In a sense, any change in one of your joints—from the base of your spine to your toe—can wrench any other part of the muscular-skeletal structure off course.

FROM MY FILES

It can be surprisingly easy, once the source of the pain is identified, to correct a mechanical gait problem that's causing both foot and back pain.

Ben, thirty-five, had lived for years with a rare neuromuscular disease that rendered one leg more than an inch shorter than the other. He suffered from intense pain in his foot, leg, and back and had also developed an overlapping toe as a result of the greater pressure he had placed on his shorter leg. Since the discrepancy was too great to be remedied with an ordinary orthotic, I made a special lift for the outside of one shoe that completely evened out Ben's gait. Such problems aren't as unusual as you might think. Millions of polio survivors, now in their fifties and sixties, have some degree of limb discrepancy because of the muscle atrophy suffered when they were stricken with the disease in childhood. Sometimes, when the difference is much less obvious than Ben's, these former polio victims have no idea why walking is so painful. A good podiatrist or orthopedist will study your gait carefully if you're complaining of both back and foot pain.

Smaller limb length discrepancies, or pain caused by arches that are too high or too low, can be remedied even more easily with a custom-made orthotic, heel cup, or metatarsal pad. These small mechanical corrections, in conjunction with standard lower back strengthening and stretching exercises, can work wonders relatively quickly. If you've been treated for chronic lower back pain but no one has looked at your feet, I urge you to see a podiatrist as soon as possible.

SELF-CARE AND PREVENTION

■ Whether you have chronic back pain or occasional flare-ups, make sure that you regularly have excess callus formations and corns removed. Routine podiatric care is more important for you than it is for other people, because you need to take special care to maintain an even walking surface on your soles and heels.

■ Doctors used to believe that rest was the only cure for back pain, but it's now widely recognized that regular exercise is essential. You'll need special back exercises, but most rehabilitation specialists will urge you to begin an overall strengthening and conditioning progam (often one that involves fitness walking). I describe such a program in Chapter 28, "The Well-Exercised Foot," but you should consult your doctor or physical therapist about the right exercise routine for you.

A SPECIAL TIP FOR WOMEN . . .

Your back will thank you if you avoid high heels. If you have a bad back, anything that destabilizes you—as high heels do—places more pressure on the muscles and encourages them to go into spasm. And, as I've already mentioned, new research suggests that high heels contribute to arthritis in the knees as well as the forefoot. Many women who habitually wear heels two inches or higher notice an immediate decrease in lower back pain when they cut their heel height by an inch.

PART IV

Foot Care for Every Lifestyle

21

The Beautiful Foot

Here comes the lady: O! so light a foot
Will ne'er wear out the everlasting flint.

—Shakespeare, *Romeo and Juliet*

Women's feet have always been associated with beauty and sensuality as well as with their obvious practical function. The idealized attributes of the female foot include lightness (Romeo would never have fallen in love with a heavy-footed Juliet); slenderness (from ankle to toe); whiteness of skin (in Western societies); smallness (remember Cinderella's ugly stepsisters, with feet too big to fit into the glass slipper?), and a conventional shape unmarred by bony bumps.

Of course, a great irony in the history of foot fetishism is that measures taken to make the feet look smaller—Chinese footbinding being the best-known example—were often responsible for ugly bone deformities. Men, it must be said, have sometimes gotten in on this act. Shoes with long, narrow, pointed toes were first popularized in England in the twelfth century by King Henry II, who—it was whispered at the time—invented them to conceal his own badly deformed toes. It seems just as likely to me that the shoes were responsible for the monarch's twisted forefoot.

Since the eighteenth century, though, the appearance of feet has been largely a woman's concern. As many serious historians of fashion and sex have noted, the effect of high heels is to make a woman look more sexually available by creating an "extended leg." In plain English, the higher the heel, the more your pelvis must tilt forward to compensate for the shift in balance that occurs when the arch of your foot rises several inches off the ground. Of course, most of us aren't consciously going for an "extended leg" when we pick out dancing shoes with stiletto heels and open toes. We just want to look good—and what looks good to us when we're in a mood for fun and romance is the image of airy sensuousness created by high heels. That biological programming may influence our brain's notion of a desirable-looking foot is hardly surprising. After *Homo erectus* decided to walk on two legs, the female of the species must have risen on her toes in the first extended-leg mating dance.

Yet styles of beauty in feet—as in every other aspect of feminine appearance—are always changing. In recent years, one of the most obvious trends is a growing acceptance of big feet. I think the admiration of girls for high-profile female athletes— most of them taller and with longer than average feet—has something to do with this change in attitude. Who could imagine those gorgeous tennis stars, Venus and Serena Williams, running around the court on Cinderella-size feet? In my practice, I also see a greater appreciation of the many ethnic styles of American beauty. I have many patients who are women of color, and "whiteness" is obviously not one of their standards for beautiful feet. In fact, the loss of dark pigmentation in spots on top of the feet is a cosmetic concern for African-American women as they age. I have one patient who models shoes for a living—you've probably seen her elegant cocoa-colored feet and calves in fashion magazines—and her main worry is that age-related skin changes will affect her smooth pigmentation.

By the way, she wears a size 10 shoe, which would have been considered unfeminine and unattractive a generation ago.

One thing that hasn't changed is the general attitude toward wide feet like mine. It's fine to wear a size 10 if it's a 10A or B, but many women won't own up to wearing a 7C. (My grandmother's generation called these "peasant feet.") When patients say they hate their feet, they're frequently talking not about deformities like bunions but about the basic inherited shape of their bones. Pedicures are often a way of consoling ourselves for what we can't change about our feet by changing what can be changed—the color and appearance of nails. Polished toenails, like lipstick, are part of a woman's beauty image not only to the outside world but also to herself. Especially in winter, when feet are rarely displayed in public, a meticulous pedicure is a sign that a woman cares about herself inside and out, regardless of whether anyone else gets to see her feet.

Because the way their feet look is often as important (or almost as important) to my female patients as the way their feet feel, I'm prepared to do anything I can to promote beauty along with podiatric health. This isn't as uncontroversial a position as you might think. Some medical professionals, for instance, oppose any aggressive treatment of nail fungus unless the nails are actually itching or infected. I don't agree. I've seen too many cases of untreated nail fungus that did metamorphose into nasty infections. But even if that doesn't happen, I don't see any reason why a woman (or a man) should put up with thick, discolored, unsightly nails if something can be done to get rid of the fungus.

In my view, there's no difference between treating nail fungus and treating facial acne, except that feet are usually covered up. And no one should be embarrassed about seeking medical help for these conditions. One of my patients, in her early twenties, walked around for six months with nail fungus because her boyfriend had said, "I can't believe how vain you are," when she suggested that they both see a podiatrist because their nails seemed to be turning green. She finally decided to get rid of both her fungus and the boyfriend.

Also, I've found that concerns about appearance and foot health generally go together. A woman who has put up with a painful bunion for years will come in because, for whatever reason, she can't stand the way it looks any longer. "I suddenly see my mother's swollen feet at the end of my legs," said one forty-eight-year-old, "and I hate that." In fact, this patient's feet felt as bad as they looked. The real reason she needed to have her bunion removed was to end the pain, but what brought her into a doctor's office for treatment was her desire to look better and fit into pretty shoes once again.

The beautiful foot is, first and foremost, a pain-free foot—and my patients want their pain-free feet to be as beautiful as possible.

WHAT MY PATIENTS WANT TO KNOW

I love to have a pedicure at the beauty parlor, but I'm afraid of getting some kind of infection. Do I have to give up professional pedicures?

No—but you do have to take extra sanitary precautions. As I've already indicated, the only way you can be sure of a sanitary pedicure is to bring your own instruments, along with disinfectant for foot basins. It won't protect you to insist on your own nail scissors if you dunk your feet in an unsterilized basin already used by a customer with warts.

Even in beauty parlors with high standards of cleanliness—and who would have her hair washed or her nails polished in an establishment that looked dirty?—there's a risk of contamination during any procedure that might lead to bleeding or that involves fissures in the skin. Beauty parlors, and nail parlors that specialize in manicures and pedicures, are incubators for all manner of fungal, bacterial, and viral infections.

I'm not talking about AIDS, though it's theoretically possible that HIV (which causes AIDS) could enter your body through a bleeding fissure in your heel. As far as I know, there's never been a documented case of AIDS being transmitted in that fashion. But hepatitis, also caused by a virus, is much more common in the general population than AIDS. I don't want to take a chance, however small that chance might be, of contracting hepatitis as a result of a pedicure under nonsterile conditions.

There's no doubt in my mind that many, many people develop warts, athlete's foot, or nail fungus after professional pedicures. I can't remember a patient with nail fungus who didn't work out at a gym, have her nails done in a salon, or both. Even more disheartening are the patients who, after lengthy and successful treatment for warts or nail fungus, turn up with a new infection. Usually, they admit under questioning that they finally thought it was "safe" to go to a nail parlor once again. (More than one of my patients has remarked that I sound like an interrogator in a spy movie when I'm on the trail of a pedicure-caused infection. *We have ways of making you talk.*)

In addition to bringing your own instruments, it's important to stick to a salon where you've observed high standards of cleanliness over time. Go to the same manicurist if possible. Have a pedicure before you go away on a trip, and you won't need another one until you get home. And never—I mean *never*—allow a manicurist to use a razor or other sharp instrument on your corns or calluses.

I love nail polish, but my nails are turning yellow. Should I care?

That depends on whether you ever want to go without nail polish again. To be serious, long-term use of nail polish and polish remover does seem to yellow the nails. If you're concerned that you might have a fungus, consult a podiatrist. I love nail polish myself and wear it most of the time, but I think it's a good idea to remove the polish and let the nails "breathe" for a day between pedicures. Most of us make our pedicures last much longer than our manicures; maybe that's why fingernails seem much less prone to discoloration than toenails. All in all, nail polish is one of the most guilt-free pleasures imaginable. It doesn't cost much, it's not fattening, and the sight of it cheers us up when we're tired, overworked, and stressed-out.

Just one caution: Don't use nail polish if you have a cut or infection in the area of your toenail. If you want to stop using polish and go natural, there are some highly effective nail whitening agents (I mix one for patients in my office). If you're being treated for nail fungus, ask your podiatrist if it's all right to use a nail whitener at the same time.

I'd rather give myself a pedicure at home, but I always make a mess of it. How can I get a professional look without going to a nail parlor?

I love this question. As you might guess, I'm a great fan of safe, at-home pedicures. It takes practice to learn how to do it properly, but, in all modesty, I must say that I'm an expert. Here are my tips for a perfect self-administered pedicure:

- If you're going to use polish, don't do it just before bed. Even if the polish doesn't smudge, sheets somehow dull the gloss if you don't wait at least forty-five minutes before climbing into bed.

- Soak your feet in lukewarm water and white vinegar for several minutes, then dry them thoroughly, especially between the toes. Wet nails are more likely to tear when you cut them.

- Cut your toenails straight across. Use a clipper with a straight edge rather than a curved scissors, and never cut nails with tiny cuticle scissors. The scissors will grow dull, and the nails will be ragged. Leave the nails closer to the tips of your toes than to the nail bed; if you cut them too short, they are more likely to grow into the skin.

■ If you have heavy calluses, try this home remedy. Mix into a paste 1 cup of kosher salt, 8 tablespoons of mineral oil, 1/2 cup of Epsom salts, and 1 tablespoon of baking soda. Apply the paste to all of the most callused spots on your foot, put the entire foot into a plastic bag, and wrap a warm towel around everything. Sit still for ten minutes, unwrap your foot, and use a pumice stone on it. (If you don't have enough time, skip this and attack the calluses another day.)

■ Apply a touch of mineral oil or baby oil to your feet before you begin polishing. The oil will sink in while your polish is drying.

■ Push your cuticles back gently, but don't try to cut them.

■ If you have any inflammation in the cuticle area at the sides of your toenails, apply the polish in a slightly narrower swathe than the bed of the nail. (This also creates the optical illusion of narrower, more elegant-looking toes.)

■ Your pedicure will last longer if you use a base coat before applying color.

■ Always clean your own instruments with soap and water when you're through using them.

■ Enjoy the way your feet look. This whole routine takes about sixty-five minutes—twenty minutes to apply and forty-five minutes to dry. Don't have the time? Your family won't leave you alone? This is as good an excuse as any for sacred private time. You deserve it. You need it.

What can I do to improve the appearance of my nails without going through a full pedicure routine?

Some people just aren't going to take the time to give themselves a pedicure, but they're still distressed about the appearance of their nails, especially if the nails have grown brittle and started to thicken. One shortcut is simply to wash your feet and slather your toes and nails with whatever lotion or cream you use on your hands. Then clip the toenails and gently push back your cuticles; it's much easier to cut brittle toenails if they've been moisturized. Do this once a week, and you'll improve not only the appearance but also the health of your nails. You'll be much less prone to cuticle and ingrown toenail infections.

I can't seem to get rid of the cracks in my heels. Is there anything that really works?

This is a classic example of a combination beauty/health issue. Heel fissures not only look bad and tear your panty hose, but they can become infected. The key to getting rid of fissures for good is routine maintenance: You can't expect to use a cream for a few days or a month and have smooth heels forever.

A great many commercial products with 20 percent urea cream are highly effective, but you need to use them every day. I've developed a copper-based cream—a formula similar to that used in hospital emergency rooms—for patients with severe fissures. There is also a new, nonprescription heel and elbow cream, containing glycolic acid, that works wonders on fissures. Ask about it at your drugstore. And as I've mentioned, I consider ordinary petroleum jelly a highly effective agent against heel cracking and inflammation. Many women abandon creams that work because they're also greasy, and no one wants to put a greasy foot inside panty hose or socks. Try creaming your feet after a bath and putting socks on just before getting into bed. The older you are, the more cream you'll need to keep fissures under control.

If your fissures are already inflamed and/or infected, you need to have them treated medically before you start using cosmetic moisturizers. Never put ordinary moisturizer on a bleeding crack in the heel.

What can I do about unsightly varicose veins on my ankles?

This is a major cosmetic concern of many women in their late thirties, forties, and fifties. It's important for you to understand that there's a huge difference between large varicosities—which may be connected with serious systemic circulatory problems and can be treated only by a vascular surgeon—and tiny reddish spider veins. The latter are broken capillaries, unrelated to any larger problem and lying close to the surface of the skin.

If a patient asks me what can be done about spider veins, the first thing I do is administer a Doppler ultrasound test to determine whether there's any involvement of the larger veins. Ultrasound actually measures the rate of blood flow to the feet: If I detect impaired circulation, I refer the patient to a vascular specialist. For these women, broken capillaries shouldn't be the main concern.

But many women do develop an unsightly network of capillaries on their ankles even though they have no large varicose veins, no history of vascular problems, and a perfectly normal ultrasound. Spider veins can be treated with a prescription vitamin K cream (which seems to improve the appearance slightly but doesn't get rid of the capillaries themselves).

The most effective way to reduce the prominence of these veins is with a high-tech laser machine (it's become available in doctors' offices only during the past few years) called the Versa-Pulse 500 or with the "cool touch" Laser 1320 NM.

Lasers can help remove a variety of abnormal or discolored tissue growths—as I've noted, they are extremely effective in treating warts—by emitting a pulse of light on a wavelength absorbed *only* by a particular pigment. The wavelength for warts, for example, is different from that used on spider veins. In all cases, the laser pulses create a thermal injury that eventually causes the abnormal tissue to disintegrate altogether or become much less noticeable. (Lasers are also used now on surgery inside the body, to break up kidney and gallstones, for example.)

Some patients say that "hits" with the laser feel no worse than a mosquito bite. Others describe each laser pulse, which lasts for a fraction of a second, as feeling like a rubber band being snapped against the skin. In most cases, we use sclerotherapy (injections of various substances that encourage the disintegration of unwanted tissue) in conjunction with the laser treatments.

The downside of laser treatment is the price tag: $500 for a fifteen-minute session (the cost varies throughout the country). Most patients need several sessions before the veins are thoroughly "zapped." And since capillary removal is generally regarded as a purely cosmetic procedure, insurance policies don't ordinarily cover it.

The upside is that the laser-treated area, after the inflammation from the procedures has subsided (this can take several months), truly restores the skin to its original appearance. Denise, forty-two, came to see me after a web of varicosities appeared on both of her ankles during a difficult pregnancy. Her circulation was perfectly fine, but the network of capillaries was so dense that she looked like she'd been tattooed. In fact, she made an appointment with me after a business associate, noticing her in sheer hose at a meeting in Florida on a 95-degree day, rudely asked if she had a tattoo. "I couldn't wear opaque stockings with the sun beating down," Denise explained. "Am I supposed to wear black stockings on the beach for the rest of my life?"

Denise was one of my first patients to try the VersaPulse, and it took three sessions to get rid of the capillaries. But today her feet do look perfectly normal—and they've stayed that way for more than three years. As is often the case, Denise's problem was medical as well as cosmetic. She had extremely loose ligaments, and her ankles constantly rolled inward, which probably made walking during pregnancy unusually difficult and contributed to the sudden emergence of varicosities. After the spiderweb disappeared, I advised Denise to wear lower heels and fitted her for a prescription orthotic to stabilize the ankle.

Laser treatments for spider veins in the foot and ankle, as well as on other areas of the body, are available in the offices of many dermatologists and plastic surgeons as well as podiatrists. If you choose to consult a cosmetic surgeon about this new laser technology, make sure that he or she is board-certified in his or her specialty and is a member of the American Society of Plastic and Reconstructive Surgeons. And the laser should never be used on your feet and ankles unless an ultrasound has ruled out a larger circulatory problem. You should definitely consult your regular doctor before going ahead with any laser procedures—for cosmetic or medical purposes.

You always see pictures of ugly red corns in ads, but I have dark brown skin and my corns are white. When I use corn pads, the corns turn whiter and stand out even more on my feet. Is there anything I can do to pare down the corns and get back to my normal brown skin color?
Corns on African Americans do look different from the same bumps on Caucasian skin; in fact, some women of color don't realize that they have corns because their sore spots bear very little resemblance to the images typically presented in ads for popular corn-removing products. While there are now many lines of cosmetics designed specifically for women of color, the best-known over-the-counter preparations used to remove corns and calluses are formulated for Caucasian skin. Unless you've found a product that's formulated specifically for women of your skin color, you probably won't get good cosmetic results.

I've used the new laser technology on a number of my African-American patients. The results have been outstanding; I've been able to remove lesions without leaving noticeable scars or significantly altering the pigmentation. I recently performed laser surgery on a black woman in her twenties who had developed excruciatingly painful and unattractive corns as a result of hammertoes. Six weeks later, you couldn't see where the laser had been used.

This is a tremendous advance—and not only for minor cosmetic procedures—because blacks are much more prone than whites to develop dense, thick scar tissue, called keloids, as a result of surgical incisions. Such scarring is always unsightly and can be painful, especially on weight-bearing parts of the foot. Regardless of what color you are, the skin on the bottom of your foot is too thin and sensitive for laser surgery. On other parts of the foot, the laser has medical advantages for people of every skin color and particular cosmetic advantages for African Americans. In general, the darker your skin color (this is true of dark-skinned Caucasians as well as African Americans), the more likely you are to develop keloids after surgery. If you've had a keloid in the past, you're more likely to develop another.

It's important for surgeons to do everything possible to minimize the size of incisions on people whose skin color makes them more susceptible to keloids. You and your podiatrist should discuss this potential problem before deciding what kind of surgical procedure is best for you.

There's something weird about my feet, and I feel like a freak. Is there anything you can do to make them look normal?

If you guessed that this question was posed by a teenager, you're right! There are a surprising number of hereditary and congenital foot irregularities (I won't call them "deformities," because they're not ugly) that cause adolescents extraordinary anguish. These include everything from overlapping toes to a "webbed foot," in which two or three toes fail to separate completely in the developing embroyo.

In the latter instance, the child is born with perfectly normal feet, except that there's a web of soft tissue connecting the affected toes. Young children don't worry much about this (the webbing rarely causes functional problems and is difficult to see unless you bend down and study the foot very closely), but they begin to be aware of their departure from the norm during adolescence. Teenagers, as we know, can be extremely cruel.

At nineteen, Samantha (whose mother was a longtime patient of mine) came to see me because she wanted an operation to separate her second from her third toes. Her webbed feet caused her no medical problems at all: Her only concern was the way they looked. Samantha had been ridiculed by so-called friends who had noticed the webbing between her toes on the beach, and she'd become self-conscious about undressing in locker rooms. It's easy to understand how a teenager feels when someone calls out, "Quack, quack," in a dressing room. And I suspected (though she didn't say so) that Samantha was also sexually self-conscious as a result of her unusual toes.

I had doubts about the advisability of this surgery for two reasons. My first reservation was psychological. I think it's a bad idea to perform any irreversible cosmetic procedure on someone as young as Samantha. One need only think about people who've spent thousands of dollars, and gone through several painful surgical procedures, to remove a tattoo that they acquired in adolescence. On the basis of my experience with other patients, I thought it quite likely that Samantha might come not only to accept but to like her webbed toes. My second reservation was medical: There's always the possibility that separating the toes could compromise circulation in the small blood vessels that supply the outer reaches of the feet.

I explained the pros and cons of the surgery to Samantha and asked her to take time to think it over. As it happens, I've had a number of patients with webbed toes over the years. One of these women (as I told Samantha) had confided to me that her husband, when they first made love, said he found her toes the most beautiful and erotic sight he'd ever encountered. A few weeks later, Samantha phoned and said she'd decided to keep her webbing. "I want the kind of man who thinks different is beautiful," she remarked.

The outcome of this case—a surgery unperformed and a patient who was willing to entertain the idea that there's more than one kind of beauty—was one of my most satisfying experiences as a podiatrist.

I rarely recommend this surgery because it is extremely delicate. The area between the toes has many tiny blood vessels and nerves, and only an experienced microsurgeon—not an ordinary podiatrist or orthopedist—can perform the operation. In a worst-case scenario, when the blood supply to the toes is compromised after surgery, you could eventually lose a toe (or toes). In my view, the risks greatly outweigh the cosmetic benefit.

I have fat ankles, and I've heard that liposuction can help me. Would you recommend it?

No, no, a thousand times no. Liposuction is a cosmetic surgery technique in which fat cells are actually sucked out of areas of the body (usually thighs, hips, and abdomen) that a woman considers ill-proportioned for her height and weight. Ankles are not a suitable area for liposuction (even if you'd be willing to have it done on other parts of your body), because the thickness of the ankle is determined by your inherited bone structure. Since there's very little fat in the ankle, the danger of damage to soft tissues or blood vessels is overwhelming during a liposuction procedure.

I've seen the damage that liposuction performed on "fat ankles" can do. It's hard for me to believe that any reputable, board-certified plastic surgeon would agree to perform ankle liposuction on a patient. Don't even think about finding a quack to change the contours of your solid, functional ankle. There's a great deal you can do with shoes to create the optical illusion of more slender feet and ankles. Make peace with the feet you have.

22

Shoe Savvy

The devil made me do it. One day, as I was investigating new shoe styles for this book in a famous New York department store, I spotted a pair of shocking pink suede pumps with three-inch heels and sharply pointed toes. "Suzanne," they called out, "buy me. Even if you hurt when you wear me, you'll look gorgeous. Heads will turn to look at your feet. Okay, I know you're a podiatrist, but don't you deserve some fun? Come on, don't be practical. I was made for you." And I bought those shoes—even though they came in only a B width and I need a C. As I pulled out my credit card, I told myself that I'd wear the shoes only when I was going out to eat in a restaurant and didn't have to stand up.

Sound familiar? The next day, I came to my senses after walking around my house in those darling, painful shoes. Back to the store they went, before I could talk myself into the idea that the shoes would feel better "once they were broken in." The podiatrist won out over the teenage girl in flight from brown orthopedic oxfords.

Nothing is more important, for both the health and beauty of your feet, than the shoes you wear. Let me tell you what I observed in the same store on the day of my shocking pink shoe attack. An extremely attractive woman, who appeared to be in her midthirties, was trying on pumps with four-inch heels *even though she had a broken toe*. Once her toe healed, the salesman assured her, the shoes would be perfectly comfortable. The woman bought the shoes, as her nine-year-old daughter watched with obvious envy and approval.

Another woman was trying on a pair of pumps that looked sensible—they had two-inch heels—but hurt her because there was no padding in the insole. She planned to take her new pumps to a shoemaker and have extra padding inserted. They didn't really feel right on her feet, she acknowledged, but she liked the way they looked. Another woman, in her early sixties, had wide feet like mine. She was buying a 9B (though she really needed an 8C) so that she could squeeze her forefoot into the extra space in front. Of course, she would have to find someone to stuff extra padding into the heels, since there was a large visible gap at the back of her too-long shoes. "What can you do?" she shrugged.

There's a great deal you can do. But there's no question that too many women, like those I observed during my shopping expedition, settle for shoes that don't fit properly. Part of that is the fault of shoe retailers. While a growing number of manufacturers offer shoes in a variety of widths—usually from A to E—few stores actually stock footwear in all of those sizes. The more fashionable and expensive the store, the less likely it is to carry shoes in an "unfashionable" width, anything beyond a B. I don't know what explains this, except that the slender foot is still the high-fashion ideal. Stocking only B widths is the equivalent of selling dresses only to women who wear a size 12 and under.

Sometimes, sales clerks simply lie and tell you a company doesn't make shoes in your width. The famous Italian shoe manufacturer, Salvatore Ferragamo, is noted for offering footwear in a full range of widths, yet a friend of mine, asking for a particular style in a 10D, was told by a clerk that the company had stopped making wide shoes "years ago." It took a phone call to the American headquarters of Ferragamo to find out that this was false information.

But you and I are also responsible for our "shoe problem." Many of us don't know—or don't want to know—our real shoe size. We want to believe the sales clerks who tell us that the shoes will be perfectly comfortable as soon as they're broken in. We're prone to impulse buying if we really love the way a shoe looks, and the salesmen know it. How many times have you been talked into buying shoes shoe a half size too small or too large because your true size wasn't in stock, and you just couldn't bear to pass up the adorable things? You still have those shoes in the back of your closet, don't you?

THE EDUCATED CONSUMER

To become an educated consumer, it's important to know something about the way shoes are made—and why certain styles are harder on your feet than others. Every shoe style is manufactured from a specific last, a plastic or wooden model of a foot, over which material is stretched to create the form. You've probably noticed that some brands never feel good on your feet, even though the shoe is the "right" size and looks like it ought to fit. That's because the last simply isn't right for your bone and tissue structure. Shoe lasts are based on each manufacturer's profile of an "average" customer; that's why international companies use different lasts in the United States, Europe, and Asia.

The average American woman has a bigger-boned, wider foot than the average French woman: Hence, the B width sold in France is generally narrower than the B sold in America. (In

Europe, many stores advertise the availability of "American" lasts to attract tourists as customers.) If your feet are much wider in front than in back (as are many women's), look for shoe catalogs that advertise "combination lasts," meaning that the master form for the back of the shoe is narrower than the form for the front.

Finding a last that suits your particular foot is the first step, but you should also check out several other features.

■ The *sole*, obviously, is the outer layer on the bottom of the shoe. Whether they're made of leather, rubber, crepe, or microfibers, soles should have some padding and, above all, should be flexible in the forefoot. At the same time, a well-constructed shoe should have a rigid shank in the middle area that supports your metatarsal arch. If you pick up a shoe and the sole doesn't bend at all from heel to toe, you'll never be comfortable. That's true whether the sole is made of highly polished, unbending leather, rigid plastic, or wood. Remember, look for a flexible forefoot and a rigid midfoot shank.

■ The *insole*, the layer of padding inside your shoe, is as important as the outer sole. Look for cushioning, especially a soft buildup in the arch area. If the inside of the shoe feels absolutely flat, that means there's no cushioning for your arches. Leather insoles add to the cost of a shoe, but synthetic materials, which don't allow your skin to breathe, encourage excessive sweating and foot odor. Feel the insole area for seams and careless stitching that may irritate the skin of your foot.

■ The *toebox* is the reinforced area around the shoe's tip. This is supposed to protect your toes but may, if improperly shaped, scrunch them together painfully. Toeboxes come in three basic shapes—round, square, and pointed. Pointed toe-boxes are hardest on feet. At the end of the twelfth century, King Richard the Lion-Hearted's knights began wearing sollerets—shoes with long, downward-curving pointed toes— to keep their feet from slipping out of the stirrups. These shoes didn't hurt because the point began only where the big toe ended.

Square and round toeboxes are equally comfortable on most feet. Square toeboxes actually conform most closely to the shape of the forefoot, and they've come back into fashion in recent years.

■ The *upper* is the top of the shoe. What's most important is that the upper not chafe any part of your foot. Leather, again, is the most desirable material from a comfort standpoint. Vinyl and polyurethane are often used for the uppers of less expensive women's shoes, but they're extremely uncomfortable to wear indoors all day. I think you're better off investing in one good pair of leather shoes—especially if you wear pumps at work—than in several pairs of cheaper shoes made of synthetic materials.

■ The *heel counter* is the reinforced part of the shoe at the back of your heel, and it helps to stabilize your ankle. Flimsy heel counters—especially in high-heeled shoes—are often the culprits in women's ankle injuries.

■ The *heel*. Whatever height or type of heel you choose, you should have a shoemaker add nonskid rubber pads to the bottom.

WHAT MY PATIENTS WANT TO KNOW

Do I have to give up high heels to get rid of my foot pain?

No, but you do need to spend less time in the heels.

First, figure out what heel height is most comfortable for your everyday pumps. Most experts say that the ideal shoe, from the standpoint of comfort and stability, has a heel between three-quarters and one inch. I recommend that you wear the lowest heel you find comfortable, as long as your shoes aren't entirely flat. As I've noted, flat, uncushioned shoes are extremely hard on adult arches.

Some women—especially those who have worn much higher heels for most of their lives—find that a one-and-a-half-inch heel is most comfortable for everyday wear at work. You may have tight calf muscles and a foreshortened Achilles tendon as a result of wearing very high heels. You need to reduce the height of your heels gradually to avoid straining those important tissues.

If your work environment permits, shift between shoes of different heel heights during the day. If it's impossible for you to change on the job, wear a pair of fitness shoes when you go out to lunch. I guarantee you'll feel better at the end of the day if you give your feet a break by changing shoes at least once.

I don't see anything at all wrong with wearing beautiful high-heeled shoes to go out for a few hours in the evening. However, I suggest that you look for dress-up shoes in the two- to two-and-a-half-inch rather than the dangerous three- to four-inch range. You'll look no less appealing in "lower" high heels, and you'll be much less likely to come home from a date with a sprained ankle.

Height isn't the only thing that counts. The *pitch* of the heel—the angle at which the heel is attached to the shoe—is equally important. From time to time, fashion designers come up with heels attached to the shoe at eye-catching, odd, and destabilizing angles. Regardless of height, the closer a heel comes to forming a right angle with the floor, the better for your feet and ankles. If you look at shoes carefully, you'll see that some of the most gifted designers have mastered the knack of making a heel *look* curvier than it really is. These shoes actually feel more steady than they appear, because the heels are carefully calibrated to provide the illusion of frivolousness and the reality of stability.

The very worst type of shoe for your foot is a high platform sandal. Platform shoes completely destabilize your ankle, because most of them lack any sort of heel counter. I've treated horrible sprains that young women suffer when the foot slips off its platform, leaving the shoe to go in one direction and the ankle in another.

I've just bought a pair of hiking shoes that look like the most comfortable shoes on the planet, and I'm in agony. How can shoes look so comfortable and cause so much pain?

I call these "faux fitness shoes," and they're among my pet peeves. There's a whole new category of fashionable footwear designed to look as if it's good for your feet—to mimic real hiking boots, or well-constructed loafers, or fitness shoes. On the inside, these shoes and boots have no cushioning and no arch supports, offering no more protection for your feet than the most insubstantial sandal. I compare these shoes to high-calorie, fat-free diet products loaded with sugar that has replaced the fat.

The best way to spot a faux fitness shoe is to put your hand inside and feel for the built-in arch supports and cushioning that you normally find in all athletic shoes. If your hand detects a flat surface, these shoes aren't good for your feet and will almost certainly hurt if you walk long distances in them. Another distinguishing mark of the faux fitness shoe is its extraordinary heaviness: Some of these cloddish-looking shoes and boots are the equivalent of the humungous backpacks weighing children down on the way to school. Unless you're planning a serious mountain-climbing trip, heavier does not mean healthier. You don't need to drag around several extra pounds on your feet when you're walking through a mall.

How do I find shoes that cover up my bunions but still feel comfortable?

This is a tough assignment that really depends on the size

and location of the bunion. In general, the worst shoes for bunions are those with pointed toes. Look for high vamps (the curve in the front part of the upper) that cover your bunion fully instead of cutting it in half. Soft material like suede is most comfortable. If you have one bunion that's much larger than the other, buy footwear in the larger size and look around for a skilled shoemaker who can help you devise inserts to fill out the loose shoe. Most of us can't afford to buy two pairs of shoes in different sizes in order to accommodate our bunions!

In fact, nearly everyone has one foot that's larger than the other. Many people make the mistake of buying the smaller instead of the larger size. It's much easier to find an insert to fill out a loose shoe than to have a tight shoe stretched. Somehow, the stretching never seems to produce the desired comfort level.

I have a closet filled with gorgeous shoes that hurt my feet. How can I stop myself before I buy more?

I gave you the answer at the beginning of this chapter. Walk around in the shoes at home, taking care to stay on the rug so that the adorable objects don't get scuffed. Live in them for an hour or two. I guarantee that if you're in excruciating pain, you won't be able to trot back to the store fast enough (in different shoes, of course) to get your money back.

For me, it actually makes more sense to buy the shoes and try them out at home than to resist them in the store and have their charms prey on my mind. I can't tell you how often I've walked out of a store without buying a pair of sensuous shoes, only to succumb the next day. The only thing to bear in mind is that sale shoes usually can't be returned. Do you think I sound like a recovering shoe addict? You're right. I understand. I feel your pain (in more ways than one).

I'm not a B width. How can I find shoes that fit?

It's easier to find shoes that match the width of your feet

today than it has been at any point since I began practicing podiatry. The rise of catalog shopping has made shoes in various widths available to women throughout the country. If you look at ads for shoes in catalogs from your favorite stores, you'll find that most of them offer quite a selection of shoes in widths ranging from AA to DD or E. Interestingly, many stores that don't stock these shoes for in-person shoppers do carry a variety of widths in their mail-order inventories.

Many women don't try these catalog offerings because, as we all know, it's impossible to tell whether a shoe fits without trying it on. But it's well worth the effort. Most national mail-order businesses make it easy to return merchandise that doesn't fit, and if you do hit on a shoe that feels comfortable, you can often order the same style in additional colors. Any woman with a difficult-to-fit foot knows that if she finally does discover a comfortable shoe, she should buy more than one pair.

Are expensive shoes better for your feet?

No. There's absolutely no correlation between price and good fit, or between price and sound shoe construction. I'll qualify that slightly: The cheapest shoes on the market are probably not as well made as those in the medium price range. It is true that leather shoes are more expensive than those made of synthetic materials, but leather itself comes in such a wide price range that nearly all women can find shoes to fit their budget. Of course, many of us justify spending a great deal of money on shoes by telling ourselves that "they'll last longer." If only it were true! The same principle applies to canvas athletic shoes. Forget about advertising and celebrity endorsements: There's absolutely no medical evidence to support the claim that shoes with famous logos last longer or are better for your feet.

I have no idea what kind of fitness shoes to buy. Help!

If you're a beginning exerciser, it can be particularly difficult to find the right shoes because you don't know how they'll feel once you're in motion. Unlike dressy pumps, these shoes can't be tested by walking around at home on the living room carpet. In general, it's a good idea to start out with shoes that don't have exaggerated features: fitness walkers or novice runners don't need athletic shoes with the deepest treads or the highest tops. As I've said, I advise the use of orthotic inserts for anyone over fifty who exercises regularly.

Here are some tips for finding top-notch *walking* shoes:

■ Choose a shoe with plenty of cushioning but medium traction. The cushioning is contained in the shoe's midsole, the area between the insole and the rubber outsole on the bottom of the shoe. Cushioning is especially important if you're going to walk on cement sidewalks or the even firmer marble floors of many suburban shopping malls open to fitness walkers in the early morning.

■ Traction is the heavy tread on the bottom of the shoe. You need shoes with more traction for higher-impact running, but too much traction for walkers can cause unnecessary resistance with each step. Your foot jams and your toes push up on the inside of each shoe, and that can aggravate existing foot problems (like bunions) or lead to new injuries.

■ The top of the shoe should be tilted slightly upward at the toe, which helps complete the natural walking stride.

■ A rise in the heel—of about one-half to three-quarters of an inch—helps reduce strain on your plantar fascia ligament and Achilles tendon. This serves the same function as a one-inch heel on an ordinary shoe.

■ Don't buy the heaviest shoes in the store. The weight of walking shoes ranges from four to sixteen ounces (a pound). Why would you want to carry around a pound on each foot?

There are much more effective and more gradual ways to increase the difficulty of your walking workout.

■ The shoe must have a firm heel counter—a stiff cup around the back and lower part of your heel that holds your heel in place and helps stabilize your ankle. The heel collar—the part of the heel counter that surrounds the top of your heel—should be well padded but not too stiff. A heel counter that's too stiff or too high will hurt and push your ankle into an unnatural position.

People who've just begun an exercise program tend to develop all sorts of unfamiliar aches and pains. Some of these may be attributable to the unaccustomed exercise, but others may be caused by the shoes themselves. For example, I've known patients who've developed lower back pain after starting to wear fitness shoes with the heaviest possible traction. Some of these shoes have an extreme "reverse shift," which means that they shift weight backward off the ball of your foot. While some exercisers find this reverse shift extremely comfortable, others—especially if they have vulnerable lower backs—find that the shift is too much for their muscles to handle. Sometimes, all you need is an over-the-counter orthotic to modify the shoe. Consult a podiatrist or a physical trainer. Be prepared to experiment.

In general, you need more traction for running than for walking. There are now many "cross-training" shoes on the market, but the only way to find out whether they're right for you is through trial and error. People who engage in a wide variety of exercises may need more than one pair of fitness shoes.

Perhaps the biggest mistake people make is not replacing their fitness shoes often enough. If you engage in any regular weight-bearing exercise more than three times a week, replace your shoes every six months. Long-distance runners should buy shoes more frequently.

How can I make certain that my shoes are the right size?

The right *shape* is as important as the right size. One way to ensure that you're buying shoes with the right proportions is to have someone else trace an outline of your larger foot while you're standing. Compare the outline with the soles of your shoes; if the outline is larger, you're probably buying a too-small size (and shoes with a too-narrow toebox). Your shoes should conform to the countours of your foot, not vice versa.

In general, as I've indicated, it's normal to wear shoes a half size to a full size larger at fifty than you did at twenty.

My shoes seem to wear out faster than other people's. Is this because there's something wrong with my feet?

Not necessarily. Any bony deformity, like a hammertoe or bunion, does place extra strain on shoes by stretching out the leather. But if you're a very active person, you may be expecting too much wear out of your shoes.

There's another possibility: You're not paying enough attention to shoe upkeep. Because I grew up in a thrifty family, I'm often surprised when I see a patient walk in wearing very expensive shoes that have worn-down heels, water-stained leather uppers, and patches on the soles that have almost turned into holes. You should be particularly careful to replace the lifts on your heels when they become worn. Uneven heels affect your gait and reduce the shoe's shock absorption.

If you're especially fond of a pair of shoes, you can extend its life by repeatedly replacing the outer sole. In many instances, a good shoe repair shop will replace the worn-out manufacturer's sole with a pad of better quality. Use shoe and boot trees to help your footwear maintain its shape. Spray your shoes with a water-repellent leather guard before you wear them the first time, and polish them regularly. Polishing shoes is another old-fashioned habit that many people have abandoned today. Polish makes your shoes feel as well as look better. By keeping the leather supple, you'll reduce chafing on any bunions and corns.

Finally, don't wear the same pair of shoes every day, especially if you have sweaty feet. Powder your shoes with cornstarch and give them a day off to breathe.

Can weight gain affect the fit of my shoes?

Absolutely, but most people don't realize this. To be sure, if you gain five pounds it won't change your shoe size. But a more substantial weight gain—of, say, twenty pounds—will affect the comfort of your shoes. Even if the fat doesn't literally go to your feet, the increased pressure—remember, twenty pounds equals thirty when you're just walking normally—will cause your feet to swell. The shoes that used to fit properly will chafe, creating new blisters and corns. It's hard for women to be honest about this with themselves, because most of us take comfort from the idea that even if we can't fit into our clothes after gaining weight, we can still fit into our shoes. I can't tell you how many patients have said this to me, and I've said it to myself. If you have gained more than ten pounds and you're not ready to take it off, be prepared to buy some new shoes in a larger size. I wish it weren't so!

23

The Pregnant Foot

Many women see a podiatrist for the first time when they are expecting their first child. And if they're like Karen, a patient of mine in her midthirties, they are often puzzled—even upset—because they've had to seek medical attention for their feet. Like so many women of childbearing age today, Karen had always exercised and paid attention to nutrition, so she was in excellent physical shape when she became pregnant. By her second trimester, though, this happily pregnant woman's sore feet were interfering with even the moderate exercise routine recommended by her obstetrician. "I expected my feet to swell up at the end of the day in the last months," she said, "but I didn't expect them to hurt every minute of every day and make me feel like I'm ninety. I'm not a sedentary person, and I just hate feeling this way."

Like many women, Karen simply didn't know (and hadn't been told by her obstetrician) that pregnancy can exact a truly hurtful—not merely aggravating—toll on previously healthy feet. During this time—when women's bodies are off balance and at their heaviest—female feet must meet the greatest challenge they will ever be required to bear in a lifetime. Most of my patients, in the course of basically uncomplicated pregnancies, ask similar questions.

WHAT MY PATIENTS WANT TO KNOW

Why do my feet hurt so much when I'm barely big enough to need maternity clothes?

During pregnancy, feet ache not only because of the extra weight but also because of the *way* the weight is distributed, even when a woman is still in her second trimester. The body's center of gravity shifts with the growing fetus, placing more pressure and strain on ligaments and muscles everywhere—especially in your abdomen, lower back, legs, and feet. During pregnancy, hormonal changes send signals to the muscles and ligaments, telling them to relax. This happens so that your uterus and abdomen will stretch to hold your baby and so that your muscles will be more relaxed during childbirth. Unfortunately, this relaxation takes place in muscles and ligaments *all over your body*, including those in your ankles and in the arches of your feet. In short, pregnancy hormones help create a temporary case of fallen arches or flat feet, one that, with proper foot care during pregnancy, will correct itself after childbirth (unlike permanent cases of flat feet caused by heredity or athletic injury).

In this flat-footed state, fatigue sets in more rapidly; you're more likely to sprain or twist your ankle, and you may develop calluses and heel pain as your new alignment puts the front, back, and sides of your feet into chafing contact with shoes that felt perfectly comfortable before your pregnancy. Dr. Scholl's recently introduced an everyday orthotic, the DynaStep, designed specifically for pregnant women.

Some women may need a custom-made orthotic insert designed to provide extra arch support in your everyday shoes.

That's what I prescribed for Karen, and she was able to resume her exercise routine and finish out her pregnancy with a minimum of foot trouble. More important, her ligaments regained their old resilience after she gave birth. If a woman doesn't pay attention to this problem during pregnancy, her muscles and ligaments may never regain their former tone—and she may wind up with a permanent instead of a temporary case of flat feet.

Proper foot care during pregnancy is especially important for the growing number of women who give birth in their thirties and even their forties. A thirty-five-year-old expectant mother is much more likely to need arch supports than a twenty-five-year-old, because pregnancy compounds the effect of ordinary age-related changes already affecting her feet.

Should I always wear flats or athletic shoes when I'm pregnant?

No. It's actually *not* a good idea to wear only flats during pregnancy, because your feet need the arch support that a low heel (about an inch) can provide. Flat shoes, by contrast, stretch out your arches even more. Many of my patients, bothered by swollen feet, yield to the natural temptation to replace their regular shoes with stretchy bedroom slippers or loose, unconstructed ballerina flats that lack any structural support. This is a serious mistake—and can lead to ankle injuries and falls—because your feet need more rather than less support while your center of gravity is constantly shifting. It's especially important to wear shoes with a firm heel counter that discourages your ankle from twisting. If your prepregnancy shoes are uncomfortable, it's smarter to invest in one or two pairs of larger, well-constructed shoes for the duration than to fall back on soft, expandable slippers that don't provide you with the support you need for safe walking while your belly is expanding.

And while well-made sneakers with a built-in arch are fine to wear while you're pregnant, don't choose thick-soled running shoes for everyday walking. They tend to have less flexible uppers and *too much traction*—something that sounds impossible. We all know that shoes with thin, slippery soles and too little traction may cause us to trip and fall. But athletic shoes with extremely thick soles (the podiatric equivalent of those humungous breakfast muffins) can also impair a woman's sense of balance. Look for shoes with medium traction—sufficient cushioning to protect the soles of your feet but enough of a connection to the ground to help you navigate at a time when your changing body affects your gait.

My advice to pregnant women is the same as my general advice on shoes: Change your shoes and shoe styles often enough (preferably, at least twice a day) to minimize perspiration and pressure on the same parts of your feet.

Do I have to take a break from my fitness routine during pregnancy?

Not necessarily. It depends on how vigorous your routine is and how well conditioned your body was before you became pregnant. Pregnancy is not the time to *begin* a rigorous fitness program, but if you've always exercised, there's no reason not to continue under your doctor's supervision. Whatever your preferred form of exercise, most doctors will advise you to diminish its intensity during your second and third trimesters.

I often suggest a fitness walking program for women who regularly run or engage in some other strenuous form of exercise and who need to switch to an easier routine during pregnancy. Walking not only keeps you in good cardiovascular shape but also strengthens the slack muscles and ligaments in your feet, legs, and back. By improving blood circulation, walking helps prevent varicose veins and foot cramping. (Avoid walking outdoors during extremely hot weather, though, because that may promote foot and ankle swelling.)

Ironically, the fact that so many women of childbearing age

do exercise regularly is the reason I must stress the importance of extra foot care during pregnancy. Fitness routines, after all, are a common cause of foot and ankle injuries—even when your muscles are strong and your body is not off balance. If you work out, avoid routines with a high impact on your foot and ankle, such as running, jumping, and hard stepping. Be especially careful about turning your ankles. Even if you're limiting yourself to fitness walking, do your workout on a level, nonslippery surface. And make sure that your exercise shoes are in top condition. I recommend buying new fitness shoes at the start of a pregnancy and again during the fifth month. Remember, your shoes will wear out faster because you're steadily gaining weight.

What can I do about swollen feet and ankles?

Avoid wearing panty hose and other tight stockings. Instead, switch to support hose, which now come in a variety of attractive colors and fashionable styles. (They're not your grandmother's ugly support hose.) To aid circulation, put your feet up frequently, especially in the late afternoon and evening. If you change to slippers at home because of the swelling, make sure that they have no-stick soles.

In addition to putting your feet up frequently, soak them every evening in cool—not ice-cold—water. (Too-cold water impairs circulation.) Then dry them carefully to discourage fungal infections, which are more common during pregnancy than at other times (probably as a result of hormonal changes affecting the immune system). Massage your feet and lower legs daily. Start with each foot and work up, rubbing the ankle, then the calf. This is most effective after a soak, when inflammation has receded and muscles are relaxed. Massage not only eases the swelling but also relieves foot cramping.

If it becomes hard for you to reach your feet in the later months, ask someone else to massage them for you. Or roll your feet back and forth over a rolling pin or an empty bottle turned sideways. Some body-care stores sell small "foot rollers" designed specifically for this purpose.

Finally, remember that the hormonal changes associated with pregnancy make your skin drier everywhere on your body, including your feet. Take particular care to use rich moisturizer cream on your heels in order to prevent cracks and inflammation.

Can nail polish hurt my baby?

No. Healthy nails form a barrier protecting your skin and preventing the absorption of harmful chemicals into the body. But it's not a silly question, because pregnant women—due to their greater vulnerability to infection—should be especially vigilant about sanitation in beauty parlors. Expectant mothers are well advised to reserve any shaving of corns or calluses— even with their own instruments—for a sterile medical setting. Even the best commercial pedicures sometimes result in the removal of a tiny bit too much skin or nail, creating a portal for infectious bacteria and viruses. You don't want to take that chance while you're pregnant. Limit your pedicure to noninvasive massage, soaking, buffing, and polishing, and you'll be pampering your feet, body, and mind. Even if you can't bend over far enough to reach your feet, it may give you a lift—and take your mind off your swollen ankles—to know that your nails are decked out in Paint-the-Town-Pink.

Should I avoid foot surgery during pregnancy?

During the later stages of pregnancy, it's not a good idea to have any type of foot surgery, or even more minor nonsurgical procedures requiring a recovery period, because you don't want to do anything to further limit your mobility while you're adjusting to a constantly shifting center of gravity. Also, you should avoid antibiotics during pregnancy unless they're absolutely necessary, so you don't want to run even the slightest risk of postsurgical infection that would require treatment with systemic drugs.

But it's fine to have minor conditions corrected with nonsurgical procedures during the first trimester. In fact, many pregnant women choose to have small problems such as corns, calluses, or ingrown toenails treated by a doctor at the beginning of a pregnancy so that they won't cause pain in the later stages. A corn that's completely painless when you're not pregnant can become acutely inflamed as a result of weight and balance changes in the last trimester. Your main goal in taking care of your feet during pregnancy is to eliminate any podiatric problems that can throw you further off balance than nature has already dictated.

Why do my feet still hurt now that I've lost most of the weight I gained during pregnancy? How can I get my feet back in shape along with the rest of my body?

Your feet may be the *last* part of your body to return to prepregnancy form simply because they've borne the entire load of your extra weight both before and after the baby was born. And don't forget that you're probably on your feet more—often with the added weight of the baby in your arms—than you ever were before you became a mother.

The stretching exercises at the end of this book (Appendix B) will serve your feet well when you're getting back into shape after your pregnancy. And they'll provide a necessary warm-up to a more ambitious fitness routine for the rest of your body.

You also need to take a careful look at your prepregnancy shoe wardrobe and discard shoes that are too tight. Some women—especially those in their thirties—may find that they now need shoes a half size or a full size larger. While you may have slimmed down and toned up to regain your prepregnancy dress size, a forefoot that has widened as the result of a fallen arch may simply require more room for the rest of your life. Don't fight the inevitable by ignoring tortured messages from your feet and insisting that they fit into a size 7 because that's the shoe size you've always worn. You may save yourself years of pain—and surgery twenty years down the road for deformities caused by badly fitting shoes—by admitting that you need a bigger shoe size now.

Finally, now is the time to get rid of any toenail fungus or warts that developed while you were pregnant. I don't like to treat these infections during pregnancy—even with local medication—because we simply don't know the rate at which such medications are absorbed by the mother and what effect they might have on the fetus. And warts, in particular, may disappear spontaneously within a few months of giving birth (probably because the mother's immune system has returned to normal). But if that doesn't happen, I advise treatment for both warts and nail fungus, not only for the mother but also to avoid any risk of transmitting these conditions to the baby. Washing your hands religiously, which most new mothers are told to do by their pediatricians for other reasons, will greatly reduce the chances of transmission until you're ready to begin treatment.

Remember that you should *always* check with your obstetrician before taking any prescription or nonprescription drugs—even local medication—while nursing. I never recommend systemic medication for nail fungus to a nursing mother.

24

Your Children's Feet

Parents are understandably concerned whenever they detect anything that seems abnormal about the way their children stand, walk, and run. Most of this parental worry is, happily, unwarranted: It's perfectly normal for your toddler to walk bowlegged until she's two and to develop knock-knees from ages two to four. In most instances, a small child's gait is merely a reflection of the ordinary development of bones and muscles. As your child grows and matures, the bowlegs or knock-knees will usually correct themselves. (See Chapter 2, "The Life Cycle of the Foot.")

Two birth defects do require early medical intervention. The clubfoot, so-called because the forefoot and heels are angled inward in the shape of a club, is the most significant of these abnormalities, occuring in approximately 1 out of every 10,000 births. You will be advised to consult a pediatric orthopedist or pediatric podiatrist as soon as possible, because various techniques for correcting this condition—including stretching exercises, bracing, casting, and taping—are begun in earliest infancy, while the foot is flexible. If these don't work, surgery is commonly performed during the first year, usually between six and twelve months.

As a parent, you should know that enormous progress has been made in surgical techniques that give the foot not only more normal function but also a more normal appearance. The earlier the surgery, the better the results (though such operations are never performed before three months). While parents understandably agonize over the thought of having surgery performed on their baby, the important thing to remember is that these procedures will make it possible for your child to engage in a wide variety of activities that are impossible with classic, uncorrected clubfeet. Children born with clubfeet used to be hopelessly crippled for life; they still are in areas of the world without high-level medical care.

Another, much less serious (and much more common) birth defect is called skew foot *(metatarsus adductus)*. The toes point inward, but the heel and the forefoot (in contrast to the clubfoot) are normal. Skew foot also requires early treatment that may include casts and braces, but a good outcome without surgery is more likely than in cases of clubfeet.

Fortunately, most of the children I see have run-of-the-mill problems that can easily be remedied.

WHAT MY PATIENTS WANT TO KNOW

My child's toes seem to overlap. Is this normal?

It's very common for babies to have toes that don't lie in the perfect straight order we've come to expect. Either the second toe overlaps the third toe, or the little toe overlaps the fourth toe. Approximately one in four babies has at least one pair of these overlapping toes, and you should take your baby to a podiatrist if you notice this irregularity. (An alert pediatrician will spot the condition and recommend that you see a pediatric podiatrist or orthopedist.)

Between six months and one year, overlapping toes can often be straightened by taping them in the proper position with adhesive. The taping must be done conscientiously every day, and you'll need to follow your podiatrist's instructions to the letter. While this condition can easily be corrected in babies less than a year old, surgery may be required in later life if the bones are allowed to harden in the overlapped position. Rigid overlapping toes can set a child up for a wide variety of foot problems in adolescence and adulthood.

My child walks pigeon-toed, and my pediatrician said he'd outgrow it. He's seven and that hasn't happened. Should I be worried?

Probably not, but I'd get a second medical opinion. Both extreme toeing-in and toeing-out are what podiatrists call "rotation" problems. Ninety percent of the time, children do outgrow these conditions—but if your child is in the other ten percent, there are things you can do now to remedy the situation.

One important reason to see a podiatrist is to rule out the possibility that your child's unusual gait is caused by an undetected bone deformity. X rays can rule that out, and you'll be told how to address the more common toeing-in and -out problems. One of the most frequent causes is extremely tight muscle contractions in the legs, and most doctors prescribe a special night splint—usually called a "bar"—to stretch out the muscles. Children dislike the bar intensely at first (not because it hurts but because it limits their mobility), but they do get used to it—and their gait straightens out within a few months.

You may be able to ward off future rotation problems by supervising your baby's sleeping position. In sleep, most babies exaggerate their ordinary toeing-in and -out position—especially when they turn over on their stomachs. Sleeping on the back discourages exaggerated foot positions and, more important, is recommended to greatly reduce the risk of Sudden Infant Death Syndrome (SIDS).

Also, take a close look at the way your child sits when she plays on the floor or watches television. Many (perhaps most) children regularly sit on their feet, and this forces the entire foot and ankle into an extreme in or out position. Discourage this kind of sitting as much as possible, just as you discourage walking with rounded shoulders.

Finally, extreme toeing-*out* can be a symptom of flat feet and weak arches (I was told as a girl that I walked like a duck). If that's the case, your child won't outgrow his duck walk unless the underlying arch problem is corrected. Treatment today does *not* mean wearing the kind of heavy orthopedic shoes I wore as a girl. Your doctor will probably recommend a light custom orthotic device to be worn inside your child's ordinary shoes. Orthotics are particularly important while children are engaged in weight-bearing exercise and sports. And most important of all to kids—nothing *shows*.

My ten-month-old is just learning to walk, and I'm about to buy her first pair of real shoes. What kind of shoes provide the best support?

Babies and toddlers aren't great shoe fans, and I'm not a great fan of shoes for babies unless they're needed for warmth and protection. Your baby doesn't need extra "support" to learn to walk properly; her developing muscles and bones are doing the job on their own. Remember when she first pulled herself to her feet? Chances are that she was in her crib, either barefoot or encased in soft footed pajamas. If your house is warm and your floor smooth, she can continue to walk around, either barefoot or in socks, as much as she likes.

Of course, your baby will need her first pair of shoes when she toddles outside the confines of the house. When I was growing up, most parents bought leather shoes for toddlers—soft white or brown oxford lace-ups for every day, patent-leather Mary Janes (for girls) for dress up. It was an article of faith that children's feet needed strong support; sneakers were frowned on for everyday wear.

Today, many children's first shoes are sneakers, miniature versions of the fitness shoes worn by adults. These are fine, as are soft leather shoes. If your child is learning to walk easily and normally, she doesn't need anything more than protection from the weather and sharp objects. Many parents buy high-top shoes for their children even before they learn to walk, out of the mistaken belief that their ankles require extra support. While there's nothing wrong with high-tops, a healthy toddler's ankles don't require shoring-up. And since children's shoes need to be replaced so frequently (as often as once every two months between ages two and six), high-tops are definitely not the smartest investment.

When you buy new shoes, leave one-fourth to one-half inch of space between the big toe and the end of the shoe. Check to make sure that the widest part of the shoe coincides with the ball of the foot, and buy a shoe—as you do (or should) for yourself—to fit the larger of your child's feet.

If your child takes every opportunity to pull off her shoes, chances are they don't fit properly. Check the feet for small blisters and other irritations. Even if the shoes are the right size, the style may be wrong for your child's foot.

A SPECIAL WORD ABOUT TEENS

One of the most disturbing developments in pediatric health during the past ten years is the steady drop in milk consumption, and therefore in calcium intake, on the part of children and teenagers. Calcium deficiency during the teen years, when the bones are still growing, is a major risk factor for osteoporosis—severe bone thinning that can lead to stress fractures—in women beyond menopause. Because the bones of the foot do not fully knit together until late adolescence, this area of the body is especially vulnerable. Stress fractures in the heel and toes, as I've mentioned, are often the first sign of overall bone loss in women.

Teenage girls are particularly prone to calcium deficiency because they often avoid dairy products in an effort to keep their weight down. One of the most important things a mother can do for her teenage daughter's future bone and foot health is insist that she get enough calcium every day. With the array of fat-free and calcium-reinforced products now on the market, there's no reason why even the most weight-conscious teen can't get enough calcium in her diet. As the mother of two daughters, I know it's tough to monitor what your children eat in the house, much less outside it. Here's where I believe in the power of example. If your daughter sees you drinking calcium-reinforced juice instead of nutritionally empty diet soda, that's worth more than a thousand lectures on basic food groups.

25

The Older Foot

A close friend of mine had a beloved grandmother—everyone in her neighborhood called her Mama Rosa—who died last year at the age of ninety-nine. Until the last year of her life, Rosa took a long daily walk around her old-fashioned New York neighborhood, stopping to talk with friends, children playing in the park, and shopkeepers with whom she'd done business for fifty years. Just after her ninety-ninth birthday, though, Rosa's feet began to hurt and swell. Her doctor's response was, "What can you expect at your age?" He gave her diuretics to reduce the swelling and advised her to stop taking her regular walks. Rosa tried to go on with her usual routine, but walking hurt too much, and she was told by the doctor that absolutely nothing could be done to keep her on her feet.

Within three months, Mama Rosa was dead. My friend says, "You know, they tell me her heart just gave out, that it was her time to go. And probably that was true. But I can't help but feel that she lost the will to live when she couldn't go outside anymore on her own. She died in her sleep, but I know she would have preferred to have had a heart attack and dropped dead while she was standing on her own two feet, on her way somewhere she wanted to go. I know because it's what she always said."

I didn't know this strong-willed old woman—and maybe nothing could have been done to help her at her age—but I do know that for my patients in their seventies and eighties, nothing is more important than maintaining their ability to walk. One of the stupidest studies I've ever seen concluded that the reduced activity of elderly people in nursing homes is responsible for a 50 percent decrease in foot problems. Why didn't *I* think of that? Encourage people to spend a large part of their day sitting or lying in bed, and they won't need fit feet.

My geriatric patients are determined to keep moving, and I suspect that will be even more true of baby boomers when they exceed the biblical limit (as most of us will) of "three score and ten." Seventy today is not considered nearly as old as it was only a generation ago, and baby boomers are likely to push the definition of "old" still further along in life. Today there are more than forty million Americans over sixty-five, a number expected to rise to fifty-five million by 2015.

While people definitely have more, and more severe, foot problems over seventy than they do in their fifties and sixties, the goal of good podiatric foot care is the same in old age as it is in midlife: to relieve the patient's pain and to maintain mobility. Unless the patient is gravely ill, the doctor shouldn't focus on the former at the expense of the latter. "What do you expect at your age?" is not an appropriate response to an aging patient who tells you she wants desperately to go on walking.

There are basically two categories of foot problems in people over seventy: those produced by systemic diseases, and those associated with the normal aging process. More than 15 percent of Americans over sixty-five have some form of diabetes, and the usual foot troubles associated with this disease become more acute, and require more medical care, in the seventies and eighties. (See Chapter 19, "Diabetes and Your Feet.") Whether arthritis is a disease or a normal accompaniment of aging (given that nearly everyone over seventy has some degree of osteoarthritis) is a matter of debate among medical researchers, but there's no question that the more severe your arthritis is, the worse your feet will feel. (See Chapter 18, "Arthritis and Your Feet.")

But—and I can't emphasize too much—painful feet aren't inevitable for people in the last decades of life. I have many patients over seventy who, once they've found the right shoes and a comfortable fitness routine, never turn up in my office except for problems as routine as an ingrown toenail or an infected hangnail. If you're in good general health, there's no reason why your feet shouldn't be in good shape too.

WHAT MY PATIENTS WANT TO KNOW

I have a very painful bunion and I'd like to get rid of it, but everyone tells me I'm an idiot to be thinking about surgery. Is it true that this surgery never turns out well for people over sixty?

Absolutely not. Surgical results on older patients were much more problematic when I began practicing, mainly because, as I've already explained, the instruments were so much less precise and inflicted much greater trauma on soft tissues. Also, general anesthesia poses a much greater risk to the elderly than to young adults. Now that nearly all bunion surgery is performed under nongeneral anesthesia, there's no special age-related risk for an otherwise healthy person.

Older patients who lead sedentary lives have generally learned to live with deformities like bunions (or they may have become sedentary because they didn't want to do anything about having the bunion removed). But I see a growing number of patients who want to deal with their bunions aggressively because they want to remain active. Linda, a grandmother in her midseventies who walked three miles a day with a fitness group, fell into this category. She came to me because the bunion she'd lived with for years had started to torture her with frequent bursitis flare-ups. She was often in too much pain to finish her fitness walk, and she said she feared becoming an "old lady" if she didn't do something about the bunion.

Linda had mild arthritis but no other diseases that would have made her a poor candidate for surgery. After checking with her internist and confirming that she was in excellent health, we decided to go ahead with a fractured bone bunionectomy. The outcome couldn't have been better. Like most of my patients who are thirty years younger, Linda was walking in a surgical shoe within a week. Six weeks later, she was back in Central Park with her fitness group. As a bonus, Linda was able to wear pretty shoes that she hadn't been able to put on over her bunion for twenty years (though that wasn't why she had the operation).

The point of this story isn't that older people should rush off to the doctor to have an operation performed on their bunions—since surgery isn't the first-choice treatment at any age—but that patients shouldn't be deprived of this option simply because they've passed a certain birthday. Mobility is a powerful component of both emotional and physical well-being. If a healthy woman wants to walk three miles a day at age seventy-five, there's no reason why she shouldn't have a foot operation to make that possible.

I have osteoporosis. I'm doing everything my doctor recommends, but is there anything special I can do to protect my feet?

Yes, and you should pay particular attention to your ankles, among the most fragile joints in women who've already suffered some degree of bone loss. Your shoes should have extremely firm heel counters to help stabilize the ankles and prevent a dangerous fall. Also, you should be concerned about not only the height of your heels but also about the width and depth of the surface that strikes the ground. Buy shoes with chunky heels.

For walking any distance, always wear fitness shoes with a great deal of cushioning. You may also want to add a cushioned heel insert inside your shoe.

Many fitness centers offer special programs of exercises designed to improve balance in the elderly. I strongly recommend that you participate in such a program if you're over seventy and have been diagnosed with osteoporosis. It's entirely possible that impaired balance—not bone loss—is the main cause of falls in elderly women. Be sure to ask whether any of your medications can affect your balance.

I've had heart bypass surgery, and my cardiologist has placed me on a special exercise program. But my feet are killing me. What can I do?

This is one of the most common questions I hear from male patients over sixty. You should view your rehabilitation period after heart surgery as an opportunity not only to improve your cardiovascular fitness but also to reinvigorate every part of your body.

Your feet are protesting because they probably haven't been accustomed to exercise for the last thirty or forty years. I've already discussed common conditions—sagging arches, Achilles tendinitis, heel pain—that affect people of any age who've suddenly increased their level of exercise. One (or all) of these things has happened to you, and the remedies I've suggested for people in their thirties and forties are just as good in the sixties and seventies.

One difference: Because your muscles and bones are older, you need to see a podiatrist and consult a physical therapist immediately. While cardiologists know what you need to do to take care of your heart, lungs, and vascular system, they aren't experts on the subject of what unaccustomed strain can do to your feet, ankles, knees, and back. Some doctors are under the mistaken impression that exercise bicycles and treadmills can't hurt your feet or your joints, but that's not so if you've lived an extremely sedentary life. If your feet are truly in agony, your physical therapist may be able to work out a routine with your cardiologist that continues the cardiovascular benefits while taking the strain off your feet.

But there's no reason why you can't get your feet into shape for a weight-bearing exercise routine. Orthotics are one solution, and stretching exercises are another. (See Chapter 28, "The Well Exercised Foot.") The older you are, the more likely you are to be overpronating and shifting too much weight toward the big toe. A podiatrist can also tell you whether you're wearing the right kind of fitness shoes for your feet.

It's especially important for older patients to select the right physical therapist. You want a therapist who's used to working with older people, not one whose main experience has been preparing thirty-year-olds to run marathons.

I've always used over-the-counter products to remove corns and calluses, but now they seem to hurt me. Why?

All over-the-counter corn and callus removal products have salicylic acid as their active ingredient. Even if you've used these products for most of your life, I don't recommend continuing to do so if you're over sixty-five. The reason why these products hurt now is that your skin is thinner. If your corns and calluses are painful, have a medical professional pare them down. In most cases, Medicare will pay for these procedures.

My nails are very yellow and they look almost deformed. Why is this happening now, and what can I do about it?

Thickening of the nail (onychauxis) is more common in people over 65 because the circulatory system—even if you don't have a systemic disease like diabetes—becomes less efficient. Extremely thick, yellow nails may also be a warning sign of poor nutrition, a contributor to a wide variety of health problems in the elderly.

If you've noticed a significant change in your nails recently, bring it to your primary care physician's attention. As I've noted throughout this book, many doctors never even look at their patients' feet. You should discuss your diet with your doctor or a nutritionist (many supplemental Medicare policies do pay for a nutritional consultation if it's recommended by your primary care physician). Poverty is the primary, but far from the only, cause of poor nutrition in the elderly. Many people, long accustomed to eating with and cooking for a spouse, develop extremely poor dietary habits after being widowed. An obvious change in your nails can be a wakeup call to start eating—and living—again.

For regular care of your nails, follow the routines recommended in Chapter 11, "Ingrown Toenails and Other Common Nail Problems." If you have arthritis that makes it difficult for you to bend down and take care of your own nails, see a podiatrist regularly.

In some instances, if a thickened nail is particularly troublesome, your podiatrist may recommend that it be surgically removed under local anesthetic. The base of the nail can be chemically cauterized so that the deformed nail won't grow back again. However, this procedure is not recommended for anyone with circulation problems.

The older you are, the more frequently you should see a podiatrist for routine foot and nail maintenance. Most of my over-seventy patients schedule monthly appointments.

I'm in good health otherwise, but I have extremely poor balance. My doctor has told me to wear athletic shoes all of the time, but I often feel shakier in them than I do in ordinary shoes. Is there any shoe that will help me feel more stable?

This common problem isn't restricted to the late sixties, seventies, and eighties. While cushioning is highly recommended to protect fragile bones and thinning skin on the bottom of the feet, your shoes probably have too much cushioning as well as too much traction. You need to be able to "feel" the ground beneath your feet. Like pregnant women—who also need to strike a balance between too much and too little traction and cushioning—you should avoid the thickest-soled athletic shoes.

In fact, athletic shoes may not necessarily be the best choice for walking. Low-heeled, lace-up leather oxfords, with crepe soles and cushioning inside, may provide the protection you need without the disorienting sense that you can't feel the ground.

Just as important as cushioning is a firm heel counter that stabilizes your ankle, something that may be easier to find in a leather shoe than in an athletic shoe. Experiment.

Also, it's important to carefully monitor changes in vision. Many falls occur not because of problem feet but because people simply can't see where they're going. This ought to be obvious, but a surprising number of my patients fail to connect their vision with their balance.

26

The Accident-Prone Foot: Seasonal Foot Disasters and Other Foolish Missteps

The things people manage to do to their feet are a constant source of amazement to me. Just when I think I've seen it all, someone walks in with an injury or infection I've never seen. Usually, the patient has made matters worse by trying to "operate" on herself.

Jasmine, a makeup artist for a hair salon, dropped a bottle of lotion on her foot and wound up with a tiny piece of glass in her heel (she was wearing backless sandals at the time of the accident). Did Jasmine immediately take herself off to a podiatrist to have the sliver removed? Of course not. She washed the area vigorously, which undoubtedly embedded the glass deeper inside her heel. Then she walked around for five weeks, making periodic attempts (with assistance, since she couldn't exactly see the spot on her heel where the glass was lodged) to remove the sliver with ordinary tweezers. When she finally came to see me, she was an emergency case: Her heel was swollen with pus, and I could see that the infection was already traveling up her leg. I had to anesthetize the area with a posterior tibial nerve block in order to remove the glass. I inserted a drain in the heel, and

Jasmine was on antibiotics for weeks. "But I ran the tweezers through a match flame before I used it on myself," she wailed.

This may sound funny in retrospect, but it was truly scary at the time. When Jasmine hobbled into my office on the arm of a friend, she was about twenty-four hours away from life-threatening blood poisoning. Any further delay would have resulted in her being hospitalized for intravenous antibiotic treatment. While most people don't wait as long as Jasmine, they usually wait too long to seek medical help. Removing foreign bodies from feet—and clearing up the surrounding infection—is a routine part of my practice.

Sometimes these cases aren't amusing even in retrospect, because by the time the patient finally comes to see me, she's terrified that something serious is wrong with her foot. Julia, forty-two, walked around for nearly six months with a lump the size of a small marble on top of her midfoot. She was a breast cancer survivor, and while her doctor had already told her that the lump in her foot was benign, Julia wasn't convinced. She'd been sick with worry, against all logic, that her cancer had come back and metastasized to her foot. When I opened up the lump, we found chips of glass inside. This kind of growth is called a foreign body granuloma: You may not even be aware that you have a sliver of glass or wood in your foot, but your body is building up tissue to wall off the invader and isolate it from your healthy cells.

Summer is my busiest time, and summer Mondays are my busiest days. That's when weekenders, having joyfully discarded their shoes to walk barefoot not just on sand but on asphalt, wooden boardwalks, and the dirty floors of coffee shops and ice cream parlors in resort towns, come trailing back to the city with trouble embedded in their feet. Here's a partial list of the invaders I've removed: shells, spines from many sea creatures, pieces of lobster claw, glass, shards of plastic from sandwich containers, wooden slivers, microscopic bits of gravel from parking lots, sewing needles. (I don't know why anyone brings a sewing needle to the beach, but if there's one needle in the sand, my patients' feet will find it.) The aluminum tabs from soda cans can slice a foot open as effectively as a knife. As far as I'm concerned, one of the great mysteries of life is why a woman will spend an hour giving her toes a perfect manicure and then expose the bottom of her feet to the filthy detritus of a throwaway society.

FREAK ACCIDENTS AND SELF-INFLICTED WOUNDS

Then there are the freak traumas caused by activities that are somewhat questionable for any adult beyond her twenties. Some years ago, my nurse Gretchen, then around forty, limped into the office with a cut-out shoe around a bunion that had suddenly become red, hot, and swollen. I asked her what had happened, since the last time I'd seen the bunion it was small and uninflamed. (Also, it doesn't exactly inspire confidence in patients to see a podiatrist's nurse walking around with a ghastly-looking foot.) At first, Gretchen said she didn't know: The bunion had simply swollen up "overnight" for no reason.

Finally, she confessed: She'd gone roller blading in tight boots, hadn't known how to stop, and had banged her bunion into several brick walls as a way of saving her head. Does this mean no one in her forties should ever go roller blading? You be the judge. If you're in great shape, start slowly, and wear knee pads and a helmet, you may well enjoy yourself. If you already have foot, ankle, or knee problems and your usual idea of Sunday afternoon fun is a movie followed by a pizza, I'll probably see you in my office on Monday if you've decided to inject more excitement into your life with a day of roller blading.

Last year I had to place a thirty-five-year-old man in a cast for eight weeks because he had jumped out of a window from the second story of his house and had broken his heel. No, he wasn't drunk at the time. He just hadn't thought there would be a problem, since he would be landing on grass. I reminded this man (a conservative banker in his other life) that gravity brings you down hard whether you're heading for grass or cement. He was lucky, in fact, that he didn't shatter the bone into pieces, an injury that would have called for much more complicated reconstructive surgery. (If you think there's something left out of this story, so do I. This would-be Superman was obviously trying to impress someone by flying out the window.)

Of course, there are freak accidents for which no one is responsible. Molly, a visiting exchange student from England, broke her big toe when a television set landed on her foot. Normally, I would have set the bone and immobilized it in a cast, but Molly wanted desperately to travel around the United States before returning home in the fall. So I did a manual realignment of the bone under anesthesia and strapped it tightly so that it would heal in the proper position. This was a judgment call: Since Molly was twenty-one and in good health, I thought her bone might heal without being immobilized in a cast. In the early twenties, bones are strong and heal quickly if there's no other problem. Had Molly been in her thirties, she probably would have had to settle for a cast.

While there's no way to fully protect yourself from accidents, I see many infections and injuries (Superman's bad landing is just one example) that could easily have been prevented. Foot injuries have a particularly adverse impact on your quality of life, because you can't ever forget them while they're healing. Here are my commandments for avoiding unnecessary trouble.

■ *First and foremost: Thou shalt not go barefoot in unfamiliar environments.* Walking barefoot on the sand is one of summer's great pleasures, but wait to do it until you have some idea of how well the beach is maintained. It's a good idea to keep your sandals on until you're out of parking lot range and closer to the water's edge, where you're less likely to encounter buried beer cans. When you're leaving the beach, put on shoes before you step into the parking lot. Wooden boardwalks are particularly unfriendly to the soles of your feet. If there's only one loose splinter, it's sure to find you.

■ *Never go barefoot in food-service establishments.* More and more restaurants in resort areas find it necessary to post signs declaring, "No bare feet admitted." I don't know why anyone needs to be told that: Any place where food is prepared, sold, or served is a breeding ground for fungal and bacterial infections as well as a source of sharp foreign bodies that can wind up in your feet. When I think about someone with an open heel fissure stepping on a piece of food that a toddler has chewed and then spat out on the floor . . . well, you get the idea.

■ *Wear shoes with closed toes and heels if you're working in an environment where spills and minor accidents are par for the course.* Jasmine wouldn't have wound up with an infected heel if she hadn't been wearing sandals when she dropped a glass bottle near her feet. No auto assembly line worker or operating-room nurse would show up for work in sandals, but a surprising number of other workplaces also have high rates of minor physical accidents. Schools, beauty parlors, restaurants, and grocery stores are just a few of the establishments that pose a risk to unprotected feet.

■ *Don't borrow other people's athletic shoes to try out a new activity.* Many people, invited to participate in an activity like skiing or roller blading for the first time, accept their host's offer of athletic shoes and equipment. If you're wearing borrowed shoes that don't provide proper support for your feet and ankles, you greatly increase your chance of injury.

■ *Be aware that construction work or painting in your home can leave residue that's harmful to your feet.* I've treated many cases of unusual skin allergies and infections caused by the residue of floor scraping and wall sanding. If any unusual work is being done in your home, wear shoes.

■ *If you know there's a foreign body in your foot and you can't dislodge it immediately, don't put off going to the podiatrist.* If you can see a small sliver just below the surface of your skin, there's nothing wrong with trying to dislodge it right away if you disinfect the area before and after. But you should see a professional as soon as possible if you're not sure you've cleaned out the entire sliver. Foreign objects do not "work themselves out," as many people try to tell themselves. As soon as you start walking on them, they burrow deeper into your foot. I assure you that you truly won't feel a thing when the podiatrist removes the invader, because the area will be numbed with a local anesthetic.

27

The Stressed-Out Foot: The Mind-Body-Soul Connection

Mark, a devastatingly handsome Tom Cruise look-alike in his early thirties, is a driven, extremely successful Wall Street lawyer. When I first saw him, Mark pulled off his socks—with obvious reluctance and embarrassment—to reveal deep, bleeding fissures in his heels. This was the first time I had ever seen fissures of this severity on a man; women, because of their thinner skin, are much more prone to such painful cracks in the heels. When I questioned Mark, he admitted that he was in the habit of pulling off his socks, hiding his feet behind his desk, and picking at his heels until they bled. This, he explained, was his way of dealing with the tensions of his high-pressure job—the equivalent of nail biting or smoking. I asked whether he wasn't afraid of someone catching him with his socks off. It was easy enough, he explained, to tell an unexpected office visitor that he was changing his shoes and socks to go for a workout at the gym. "Why don't you really go for a workout to get rid of the stress?" I asked. "I don't have the time" was the predictable reply.

Mark had made an appointment with a podiatrist because he

was concerned—and rightly so—about the possibility of infection. While it was easy enough for me to cushion his heels with sterile gauze and prescribe soothing creams to heal the fissures, there wasn't any easy way for Mark to change the behavior that had led to this ugly and potentially infectious condition. All I could suggest was exercise or psychotherapy (preferably both). There was something unsettling and compulsive about Mark's story, something akin to more extreme cases of anorexia nervosa and self-mutilation in teenagers.

This was the first, but not the last, time I would see vivid evidence of the toll that emotional stress exacts on the feet. In the late nineties (I don't remember many of these cases from the early days of my practice), I saw many women patients with the same kind of self-induced fissures in their heels. Because of panty hose, women can't pick their heels in their offices. They have to wait until they get home, change into their jeans, and curl up barefoot. One woman came to see me when she dried her feet after a shower and discovered, to her horror, that the towel was covered with blood.

The importance of the mind-body connection is now generally acknowledged in every area of medicine, and your foot, because it's the repository of so many nerve endings, reflects the state of your mind and heart. Stress isn't going to give you a bunion, but, in my view, it certainly does render you more susceptible to viral, bacterial, and fungal infections. I've had patients whose warts were banished for years, only to pop up once again during a job or marital crisis. When you're extremely nervous, both your hands and feet are likely to pour out great quantities of sweat. I have one patient who always brings an extra pair of socks to work in his briefcase on days when he's scheduled to make a major presentation to his boss. "If I don't change socks afterward," he confided, "I can actually hear a squish in my shoes. It's like I've been walking around in a rainstorm."

For most of us, stress doesn't translate into any specific ailment but into a general, aching tiredness in our feet at the end of the day. "Foot weary" is a good term: There are days when all annoyances and disappointments seem to concentrate themselves in our feet (often accompanied by a splitting headache). On these days, you should do something special for your feet.

Those rich nerve endings, so sensitive to your state of mind, can work for you instead of against you. Learn how to release the tension in your feet, and the rest of your body and mind will follow.

PAMPER YOUR FEET WITH MASSAGE

There's no way that I could possibly say enough about the physical and psychic benefits of foot massage. Massage is not "alternative medicine" (or "voodoo medicine," as its critics sometimes call nontraditional methods of healing). I prescribe medical massage as part of physical therapy for nearly all of my postsurgical patients. Massage increases circulation and blood supply to the injured area, relaxes traumatized muscles, and reduces swelling. Swelling, whether it's triggered by the trauma of surgery or simple overuse (if your job requires you to stand all day, for instance), pools lymphatic fluids in your feet. Massage gets those fluids moving back toward the heart and removes pressure from the nerves in your feet. All of this not only promotes healing but also lessens pain during the postsurgical recovery period.

There's no substitute for the hands-on skills of a *human* massage therapist. One of my pet peeves about health insurance plans is that they frequently refuse to pay for old-fashioned massage administered by a human being while coughing up bigger bucks for high-tech physical therapy treatments. I can attest to the fact that both technology and human skills are needed in the rehabilitation process.

If you're not injured but suffer frequently from tension, aches, and cramping in your back, leg, and foot muscles, an occasional massage from head to toe will do wonders for you. If you can afford it, look for a good massage therapist in your area. Some therapists will come to your home—an even more relaxing experience than massage in a clinic or health club.

Many beauty parlors offer massage, but I'd stick with a licensed medical massage therapist. Unlicensed masseurs and masseuses are everywhere, but state licensing usually ensures that the person who's working on you has received professional training. Ask your therapist what type of massage he or she's been trained to perform. (In Europe, where medical massage is highly respected, therapists study anatomy as well as various massage techniques. There are many schools in America that train students in Swedish massage methods. *Acumassage*, which makes use of traditional Chinese acupuncture points, is another term you'll hear.)

Physical therapy facilities generally hire only licensed massage therapists, and many of them do private work on the side. A reference from someone you know is the best, and safest, way to find a good therapist. Whatever you do, don't pick someone out of an advertisement in the "personal services" column of a newspaper. There's medical massage, and there's the kind of massage that's a euphemism for sexual services.

If you can't afford an all-body massage that includes your feet, you can give yourself a foot massage. Many of my patients' initial reaction to this suggestion is "That's too much work." But when they try it, they like it. I give myself a foot massage at least once a week.

You can receive a massage with no effort on your part by

buying one of many commercial devices that bathe, warm, and massage your feet. Vibrating fingers work on you for as long as you like, and automatic controls allow you to adjust both the heat and the intensity. But many of my patients say their feet feel better after they've given themselves a massage. That's not surprising because the human hand is far more sensitive—better able to tell us where it hurts—than any electronic device.

If you're going to give yourself a foot massage with no mechanical assistance, here's how to do it:

- Warm your feet first in lukewarm (not hot) water. I soak my feet for about fifteen minutes in Epsom salts. This dilates the blood vessels in your foot, preparing your nerve endings to be more receptive to the stroking and pampering they're about to receive.

- After you've warmed up your feet, sit with one leg crossed over the other, with the sole of one foot facing you. Some people sit on the edge of the tub (I don't recommend this, because it's a precarious posture), while others crawl into a big comfortable chair. One of my best friends reclines in a hot tub while she massages her feet. This can be very easy if you have a large tub, because the water buoys up the leg you're massaging.

- Use your thumbs as your massage tools. Move them over the sole in circular fashion; dig as deep as you can. Concentrate on small areas at a time, and work from the tips of your toes toward your heel. (You're trying to get the fluids in your feet moving back toward the heart.) As your hands move over your foot, give extra attention to the areas that feel knotted. At first, some of my patients mistakenly think these knots are tumors—but they're simply overworked muscles in spasm. It should tell you something about the tension in your feet when your muscles are so tightly clenched that they feel like large lumps.

- Turn your foot over and use your thumbs—but more gently—on the top of the foot. Pay particular attention to the toes, tugging each one gently, back and forth and from side to side, between your thumb and forefinger.

■ Switch feet and repeat the process. The entire massage, if you do it right, should take about twenty minutes. Then reward yourself with a scented bath.

Some of my patients also enjoy the extra pleasure of swapping foot massages with a partner. This is one good way to stop thinking of your feet as ugly and unsexy! The nonattention to the sensuousness of feet is definitely a relic of Puritanism in the United States. In Sweden, daily foot baths for women and men are as routine as taking showers and brushing teeth. In India, toe kisses are part of the rituals of lovemaking outlined in the *Kama Sutra*. The pioneering sex researcher Alfred G. Kinsey noted that the tissues of the toes expand during sexual arousal. "He makes my toes tingle" is more than a casual expression.

In any event, there is something extraordinarily intimate—in an emotional as well as a physical sense—about letting a partner touch your feet. Think about it. Other people touch us frequently on our arms, back, and cheeks, with gestures that range from friendly encouragement to a caress. But once our mothers stop bathing us, no one touches our feet for years. Even if toe kisses aren't your idea of foreplay, the intertwining of feet is very much a part of lovemaking—before, during, and after.

WHAT MY PATIENTS WANT TO KNOW

As I've said, I don't think there's anything "alternative" about medical massage. But many of my patients do ask me about other treatments that elicit reactions ranging from skepticism to ridicule from much of the medical establishment. I try to combine my honest skepticism, as someone trained in traditional medicine, with the open-mindedness of a professional who believes there is a role in treatment for methods not generally used in Western medicine.

I've heard that reflexology is even more effective than massage. Is there any harm in trying it?

Unlike massage, reflexology *is* alternative or holistic medicine, meaning a great many people swear by it, but there's no scientific evidence demonstrating its effectiveness.

You need to know something about the history of reflexology in America to understand how it differs from medical massage. Reflexology was introduced in the United States in the first decade of the twentieth century by William H. Fitzgerald, a medical doctor. According to Fitzgerald's theories, the body was divided longitudinally into ten zones, with each zone ending in one of the ten toes. His idea was that all of the organs lying in the same zone influence one another's well-being, and problems in one organ might be corrected by working on another organ in the same longitude.

The eye and the kidney lie in the same zone, so (if you carry reflexology to an extreme) you might expect to improve your vision by doing something nice for your kidney. Personally, I wouldn't throw away my glasses. It must be recalled that reflexology was born in an era when both doctors and the public were inclined to believe that physiognomy determined not only health but all human behavior. According to the pseudoscience of phrenology (another late Victorian invention), a criminal could be identified by analyzing the shape of his skull.

As far as the foot is concerned, reflexologists divide it not only into ten longitudinal zones but also into horizontal zones corresponding to the trunk of the body. Toes are especially crucial, because each of them lies at the tip of what reflexologists call an "energy zone." According to this notion, congestion at the tip of the zone can disrupt the functioning of every other body part in the same zone.

When a reflexologist works on a patient's feet, what he's doing looks like an ordinary massage, but he's actually trying to locate particular pressure points supposedly connected to other parts of the body. Unless you accept reflexology's basic theory of how body parts influence one another, all of this sounds far-fetched. I don't know many people who are likely to buy the theory that a sore throat can be soothed by pulling on the big toe, or a diseased liver can be helped by stimulating the ball of the right foot.

The difference between massage and reflexology is that massage lays claim only to improving circulation and reducing swelling in the foot itself. If the rest of the body feels better after a foot massage (as it usually does), that's because of the overall relaxing effect. That said, I know that many experienced reflexologists give wonderful massages. It probably won't hurt you to go to a reflexologist, but it may not help you either. There are many books on the theory and practice of reflexology, but they don't make specific healing claims. (That could get the authors in trouble for practicing medicine without a license.)

If you are seeing a reflexologist for your feet or any other part of your body, please don't use the sessions as a substitute for standard medical care. I'd give the same advice to anyone who was battling cancer and felt that she was benefiting from nontraditional healing methods such as herbal treatments. Do anything that makes you feel better, but use alternative medicine only as a supplement for therapy that's been scientifically tested and found effective.

The fact that someone says, and believes, that she was cured of cancer by herbs, or reflexology, or bathing in seaweed, or some wondrous potion no one has ever heard of is *not* scientific evidence. The patient may not have had cancer at all, or she may not have really been cured. Scientific testing, by contrast, must establish the original diagnosis beyond a doubt. Then the outcomes of different treatments are compared with one another— and with the outcome of no treatment at all. Only through this method can one type of therapy be proved more effective than another. When podiatrists began doing ambulatory foot surgery, for example, many studies were conducted to determine whether the results were as good as those obtained when patients were hospitalized overnight. Only when the results of those studies were analyzed could we assure patients that they were likely to fare better with ambulatory surgery than with a hospital stay.

What's your opinion of acupuncture as a way of relieving foot pain?

I think there has to be value to any method of pain relief that's been used as long as acupuncture has in China. As any doctor knows, there are mysterious cases of persistent pain with no obvious cause. I've seen some of these patients in my own practice and have been frustrated by my failure to relieve their anguish through conventional treatment. I do sometimes refer such patients to acupuncturists, and some have reported significant relief. I should say that in New York City, with its large Chinese-American community, there are many acupuncturists who also have medical or podiatric degrees. In my view, these practitioners have access to the best of both worlds. Around the country, a growing number of hospitals have doctors on staff who are also trained in acupuncture. If you're interested in acupuncture, ask a local hospital to provide a referral. (Some M.D.s are absolutely close-minded on this issue, so you may have to go beyond your own doctor to obtain a reliable referral.) For general foot pain, you might also try Dr. Scholl's new Magna-Energy insoles with shock-absorbing gell.

I have a bunion and it always feels worse when it rains, but I've been told that's an old wives' tale. Does the weather really affect your feet, or is it all in my head?

I guess you could call me an old wife. There's no question that humidity has a deleterious effect on many foot ailments. If you have an inflamed bursal sac around your bunion, it will tend to swell in humid weather. In my experience, that's true of almost every inflammatory foot condition. People with arthritic feet feel worse in both cold and humid weather, especially when the two are combined. Also, both hot and cold temperature extremes are terrible for anyone with impaired blood circulation to the foot.

If you have any arthritic, inflammatory, or vascular condition, you must take special care with your footwear in cold and rainy weather. You should be particular about your boots, because the wrong boots not only chafe deformities like bunions and hammertoes but also may cut off circulation. Take special care not to buy boots that hit you in midcalf, the thickest part of your leg. If the boot constricts your calf, fluid will pool in your lower leg, ankle, and foot. This is uncomfortable for anyone and downright dangerous if you have diabetes or rheumatoid arthritis. Always take your boots off at work. All boots are less comfortable than shoes, and waterproof boots are usually made of synthetic materials that don't allow your feet to breathe.

I've had horrible burning and tingling in my foot for six weeks, and tests haven't turned up any explanation. My doctor has suggested psychotherapy, but I can't believe this is all in my head. I'm really scared. How can I get someone to take this seriously as a medical problem?

Unfortunately, there are still medical practitioners (a declining number, but anyone can encounter one) who don't take pain seriously unless a definitive cause can be established through standard physiological tests. While psychotherapy can certainly be helpful when a patient is trying to cope with pain, the pain itself must be regarded seriously and treated aggressively.

When I first saw Anne-Marie, the patient who posed this

question, I immediately suspected that she had a highly mysterious nerve problem called reflex sympathetic dystrophy (RSD). RSD is a perfect example of how far we still have to go in our understanding of the role emotions play in certain diseases. This condition truly isn't well understood, but the syndrome *is* well documented. The first symptoms of RSD include burning, tingling, and numbness; generalized swelling; warmth in the foot and ankle; and bouts of severe, inexplicable pain anywhere in the foot. They may appear after a minor or major physical trauma, or they may seem unconnected to any event in the patient's life.

The main clue to a diagnosis of RSD, however, is that the pain is out of proportion to any cause suggested by test results. If a patient is feeling intense pain in her forefoot and an X ray reveals a tumor, you can conclude that the tumor is the source of the trouble. In RSD, there's no obvious correlation between test results and the severity of pain. Sophisticated tests, such as the MRI, EMG, and nerve conduction velocity analyses, may show soft tissue and nerve irregularities, but nothing to explain exactly why the patient is in such great pain.

Yet the physical progression of RSD symptoms will continue if the pain cycle isn't interrupted. After about three months, joints stiffen and the foot and leg muscles begin to show signs of atrophy. Bone density tests reveal osteoporotic changes typical of women in their seventies. And if the disease is unchecked, these changes will become irreversible.

Also—and I consider this of prime importance—it's a mistake to make snap judgments about a patient's psychological state when she comes to you for pain relief. You have no way of knowing whether a suffering patient was anxious and depressed before her pain began or whether the pain triggered her distressed mental state.

In Anne-Marie's case, I referred her to an internist whom I knew was familiar with RSD and would treat the condition as a serious threat to my patient's health. We worked along with her psychotherapist to attack the symptoms on all fronts. Anne-Marie was placed on a short-term course of antidepressants because, by the time she came to see me, she was clinically depressed. I started her on physical therapy, including gentle exercises in water that didn't add to the pain in her feet, to arrest the muscle atrophy in its early stages. In some cases, it's also advisable to use an epidural block anesthesia injection to interrupt the pain cycle. For Anne-Marie, that wasn't necessary. Her response to both antidepressants and physical therapy was dramatic, and she was able to stop taking the drugs as her pain receded.

Of course, mysterious pain is not always caused by a serious disease—but you need to check out every medical possibility. I'm certain of one thing: No patient should ever be told, by any medical professional, that the pain is all in her head. That's as ridiculous as saying, "The pain is all in your body." Pain is indivisible: It's the product of our biology and our emotions.

While I may not believe that pulling on your big toe will cure a sore throat, I am absolutely convinced that healthy, fit feet are crucial to your physical and emotional well-being. No alternative healer (or, for that matter, traditional doctor) can do for you what you can do for yourself through a well-conceived exercise program. In the next chapter, I tell how to get and keep yourself moving for a lifetime.

28

Is your idea of exercise a walk to the door to get the Sunday paper in order to crawl back into bed with it? Or are you out jogging before the paper is delivered? Regardless of how physically active you are (or aren't), strong and flexible feet are a fitness essential. You can do without beautifully sculpted biceps and triceps, but weak ankles and strained ligaments in your feet will prevent you from fully enjoying any activity.

Paradoxically, fitness fanatics are just as likely as confirmed couch potatoes to neglect their feet. I'm always baffled when a serious jogger limps into my office because she failed to stretch her Achilles tendon before a 10K run. But perhaps this isn't so surprising. It's not uncommon for highly motivated athletes (amateur and professional) to focus more on their ultimate goals—from winning a weekend tennis match to capturing an Olympic gold medal—than on the smaller physical and mental steps that can't be overlooked in pursuit of the long-term goal.

Most of us, of course, fall somewhere between the truly sedentary and the religiously fit: We move around a lot in our everyday lives, exercise sporadically, and feel guilty about not doing more to "get in shape." We're the people who buy exercise bikes, install them in our bedrooms, use them twice, and then allow them to languish as clothes racks. We read articles about physical fitness, but we resent it when anyone nags us about the need to exercise more.

I've found that all of my patients, whatever their level of physical activity, can benefit from daily foot exercises. These can also help prepare you for a more vigorous weight-bearing routine. At the very least, toning up your feet provides pleasurable soothing and stimulation for an area rich in nerve endings. These exercises are designed to expand blood flow to the feet and to minimize the soreness that signals foot fatigue at the end of the day. Best of all, foot exercises require only a small investment of time (no more than twenty minutes a day), and they don't have to be done all at once. They're easy to learn, cost nothing, and aren't dependent on some expensive piece of equipment.

Here are some of my favorite exercises. I've developed many of them myself and have garnered others from my patients and medical colleagues. Some of these don't even sound like "exercises," because you can do them while sitting at your desk or watching television. But I assure you that if you incorporate these small moves into your daily routine, you'll feel the difference in a matter of weeks. Whether you're on your feet all day at work or behind a desk, tune-up and tone-up exercises will give you a mental as well as a physical lift.

THE FOOT PRESS

While sitting on a chair, take off your shoes and cross your legs at the ankles, keeping one foot on top of the other. Try pulling your feet away from each other, putting as much pressure on them as you can. Hold the pose as long as possible, preferably for two minutes. (If you think this isn't a real exercise, you'll soon change your mind when you feel the stretch in your thighs.) Next, sit on the floor and bend your legs at the knees, pressing the soles of your feet together. (Men, with less flexible pelvic cages, have more difficulty with this than women.) Hold the pose for two minutes. Doing this exercise a few times during the day is a guaranteed stress buster as well as a muscle relaxer.

FLEXION EXERCISES

■ Place a phone book on the floor. Stand on it and curl your toes over the edges of the pages. You probably won't be able to ripple the pages at first, but you will as your flexibility increases. If your foot is tired, it's likely to feel much more relaxed after this exercise.

■ Simply roll your shoeless feet over a handful of marbles, pencils, or a small empty bottle. This stimulates blood flow to the feet and acts as a self-massage.

■ Pick up pencils with your toes for a minute or two.

■ Take off your shoes and write imaginary letters of the alphabet in the air with your toes. Write A to Z with one foot, then with the other. If you have children, they'll love doing this exercise with you.

CIRCULATION EXPANDERS

■ Lie on your back and "climb the walls" with your feet. This builds strength and is a great way to restore circulation to feet that are tired enough to feel numb. Go up and down the wall with one foot, then the other.

■ Lie on the floor on your back and lift one leg at a time into the air at least two inches (preferably more) off the floor. (The other leg may be comfortably flexed.) Draw a circle with the raised leg in one direction and then in the other, and try to keep the leg up for at least sixty seconds. If this is too difficult at first, hold the count for thirty seconds. The idea is to keep the leg above the level of your heart so that the blood flows faster back toward the heart; this exercise is particularly good for people who have a tendency to retain water around their ankles. It's also a great exercise for strengthening the abdominal muscles.

■ Take off your shoes and stretch, wiggling all of your toes at the same time. Walk across the room on your toes, then lean back and walk on your heels. This stretches every muscle from your toes to your legs and is particularly relaxing for people (like sales clerks) whose work requires them to stand for long periods in one place.

■ Slip off your shoes and pretend that you're pumping the gas pedal of your car, first with one foot and then with the other. (You can do this in your car, but put on shoes before you drive off.) Keep a pair of flat shoes in your car for driving, and your feet, ankles, and calves will get an automatic workout every time you start the ignition. If you drive in high heels, you're depriving yourself of an automatic foot-stretching workout. When you're wearing heels, the ball of your foot has to do all of the work and the rest of the muscles never get a chance. This definitely increases the physical stress of driving.

■ Rolling pin massage. This isn't exactly an exercise, but it's a way of giving yourself a foot massage to increase circulation and instantly relieve tension. Place a rolling pin under one foot, and roll it back and forth. Repeat with the other foot. Keep rolling back and forth until the soles of your feet start to tingle. Your feet will actually turn pinker as the blood flows toward your toes.

These exercises, as you can see, are simple enough to be incorporated into anyone's daily routine. I don't think there's anyone, at any fitness level, who can't do them or won't benefit from them. "Real-life" exercises also serve as a warm-up for the more demanding stretches I've recommended to guard against plantar fasciitis and Achilles tendinitis and heel pain.

Pay particular attention to Exercises 1–4, the standing calf stretches on pages 262–265. If you start doing these twice a day in your twenties—regardless of whether you engage in more strenuous fitness routines—you'll be taking a big step toward avoiding the arch and Achilles tendon miseries that plague so many people in their thirties, forties, and fifties. These exercises are also useful if you're trying to retain flexibility in arthritic feet and ankles. They can be done by people of any age; many of my patients in their seventies begin each day by warming up with stretches.

While I recommend this conditioning routine to everyone, stretches are particularly important for people who lead generally sedentary lives but engage in bursts of exercise on weekends or vacations. You're at the highest risk for soft-tissue injuries, those caused by strain and overuse rather than by a sudden, traumatic event.

WALKING: THE FOOT-FRIENDLY EXERCISE

The purpose of stretching, massaging, and generally pampering your feet is to prepare them for action, so that they'll take you wherever you want to go and enable you to engage in other forms of vigorous, whole-body exercise. When my patients are on the mend from whatever specific foot problem has brought them to my office, many of them ask me to recommend a foot-friendly exercise program. Without hesitation, I urge most of them to begin walking for fitness.

What is "fitness walking," as opposed to just ambling down the street? If you're walking for fitness, you generally have to set a pace of a mile in twenty minutes. This is easy for people accustomed to vigorous walking, but it's hard in the beginning for those who never use their feet when they can ride.

The twenty-minute mile is the rate at which walking becomes an aerobic exercise—meaning that you're moving rhythmically, continuously, and briskly enough to force your heart and lungs to work harder to supply your muscles with oxygen. By the end of a good aerobic walking workout, you'll break a mild sweat and feel slightly—but not uncomfortably—winded. Your muscles will feel pleasantly tired but not cramped. As you build up your endurance, you'll have to walk farther and faster to reach the same point. That's because your muscles and your entire cardiovascular system are growing stronger and more efficient: It takes more effort to make you breathe hard after a few months of fitness walking. Many once-sedentary walkers have told me that they used to huff and puff when they climbed one flight of stairs but they now incorporate hills and steps in their regular walking routine.

Fitness walking has been shown to reduce the risk of heart attack by cutting blood cholesterol levels and lowering blood pressure. And, because it's a weight-bearing exercise, it may also reduce the rate of bone loss in menopausal women. (Swimming, by contrast, has only aerobic benefits. Only weight-bearing exercise—movement that creates an impact between your foot and the ground—can affect bone density.) The rhythmic, continuous nature of walking makes it less likely that your feet, ankles, or knees will be injured.

Because I have treated so many runners with badly injured feet and ankles, I have a strong bias against jogging and in favor of fitness walking. The reason is straightforward: pressure on your feet of one and a half times your body weight while you're walking versus three to four times while running. I know that runners love to run: Many of my patients say they can't imagine

234

life without jogging, even though they've already injured them-selves and fully expect to injure themselves again. But I still prefer walking for anyone, of any age, who's just starting an exercise program.

Make no mistake: Fitness walking is real exercise, and you must embark upon your program gradually. You might start out by walking just twenty minutes a day, three days a week, and at a pace much slower than the twenty-minute mile at which walking becomes aerobic. Gradually increase the length, pace, and frequency of your walks over three to four months, until you're walking forty-five minutes a day, five times a week. If you wind up walking three miles in forty-five minutes, you'll *know* from the sweat on your back that fitness walking is a real exercise.

Walking is so real an exercise, in fact, that you should consult a doctor first if you're over fifty, have any history of heart dis-ease or high blood pressure, are significantly overweight, have a chronic medical condition such as diabetes or arthritis, or are taking a prescription drug that might interfere with normal perspiration. Fitness walking is of great benefit to people in all of these groups, but your doctor may set special guidelines that take your medical situation into account. In most cases, doctors are *thrilled* when a sedentary patient comes in and says she's ready to start exercising.

Fitness walking, by the way, is not racewalking, an Olympic sport characterized by straight legs, swiveling hips, pumping arms bent at the elbows, and speeds as high as eight miles an hour. You may see stiff-legged fitness walkers imitating race-walkers, but don't do it. The unnatural gait might have been invented to yield ankle and knee injuries.

If you feel any pain in your feet or legs while walking, that's a signal to stop. This is particularly common when people first embark on a walking program. Your body may not be quite ready for the pace you're setting, you may need more fluids during your walk, or you might be wearing the wrong shoes.

IF YOU CAN'T LIVE WITHOUT RUNNING

Many of my patients do run, everything from a mile a day to marathons. And while, as I've said, I don't consider running the ideal exercise for anyone over thirty, I'm well aware of the immense psychological and emotional satisfaction many runners derive from this demanding high-impact exercise. If you're passionate about running, there are things you can do to reduce the stress on your joints.

First, the stretching exercises for your Achilles tendon and calf muscles are even more essential as a warm-up for runners than for fitness walkers. Don't hurry through these exercises because you're anxious to get started on your run.

Athletes in high-impact professional sports now realize that the durability of their joints depends in large measure on the strength of the muscles around them. Look at the well-developed thigh muscles of major-league pitchers, and you'll see why their knees and lower backs are able to absorb the weight of their powerful follow-through after each pitch.

If you're going to run regularly, you'll need to work on strengthening your thigh muscles and hamstrings so that they can provide protection for your ankles and knees. This kind of conditioning is tough, and you should begin under the supervision of a therapist or physical trainer. Rochelle Rice, a personal trainer who has worked with many of my postsurgical patients, points out that if you're just beginning to run to improve your cardiovascular fitness, your muscles aren't yet ready to do all of the strengthening and stretching exercises recommended in popular exercise books. Don't try to do it on your own if you don't have exercise experience.

I can't stress enough that you should have a complete physical—including a cardiac stress test if you're over forty—before you begin a running program. There's no one-size-fits-all running regimen (or, for that matter, any other exercise routine). "Begin slowly" is good advice for anyone, but that means something different for a thirty-year-old with no health problems, a forty-five-year-old with high blood pressure, and a sixty-year-old with arthritis.

Above all, you need to pay attention to what your body is telling you if you feel pain during or after your run. Mild pain at the start of your run means that you need to increase the length of your warm-up. If the pain disappears after you've been running for a few minutes, that's a dead giveaway that your muscles weren't loose enough to start. By warming up your muscles at high speed rather than through gentle stretches, you're making them do double duty—and they're likely to rebel sooner rather than later.

If your pain *increases* during your run, cut back immediately on your speed and distance. If the pain then disappears, you can slowly start to increase your distance again in a few weeks. If you've had pain, I'd suggest that you give yourself several weeks of painless running before you try to do more again. If the pain recurs, see your doctor. And stop running right away if you have any pain that doesn't disappear after you've rested.

Finally, be sure to take time to cool down with stretches, followed by a warm bath or shower. Your muscles need to shift gears at both ends of your run. Runners say their daily routine leaves them feeling both relaxed *and* energetic—a combination that goes a long way toward explaining why so many people won't consider giving up running even when it's taking a toll on their joints. In order to obtain that pleasurable runner's "high," you must allow enough time for your body to adjust. Pain, whether it comes during or after a run, is definitely not a high.

WHAT MY PATIENTS WANT TO KNOW

I have painful arthritis in my ankles and feet. Are there any exercises that will help?

All of the gentle stretching exercises I've described in this chapter, along with the more demanding stretches in Appendix B, will help maintain flexibility in arthritic foot and ankle joints. I'm assuming that you've had a rheumatological workup and that you're receiving the best possible medical treatment for your particular form of arthritis. It's now well known that regardless of when arthritic symptoms first appear, moderate exercise seems to diminish pain in patients of all ages. It's a clear case of "use it or lose it."

But the key word is "moderate." Degenerative osteoarthritis becomes more common and intensifies with age, but it's really related more to the demands that have been made on the joints than to the number of birthdays you've celebrated. Wayne Gretzky, the fabled Hall of Fame hockey player who retired last year at age thirty-eight, became a spokesman for the Osteoarthritis Early Awareness Campaign when he was diagnosed with degenerative arthritis in both of his shoulders (too many collisions with the boards during a twenty-year career). Gretzky is hardly inactive: He plays thirty-six holes of golf a day. And that's an excellent example of the kind of adjustment anyone with arthritis must make. Tennis, which requires you to lift your arm over your head, would not be nearly as good a sport as golf for anyone with shoulder arthritis.

Swimming, because it places no pressure on the joints, is highly regarded as a beneficial exercise for all forms of arthritis. Most of my patients with degenerative arthritis in their feet and ankles don't have to give up weight-bearing exercise, but they do have to scale it back. Joggers, for example, should either cut down on distance or switch to brisk walking. Singles tennis players should switch to doubles (or to golf or cycling).

The emotional and psychological willingness to make the adjustment is the key to coping successfully with arthritis. I've observed a vicious cycle in which a hard-driving type A exerciser develops arthritis in the early forties but refuses to acknowledge what's happening (or to listen to the podiatrist who tells him that running ten miles a day is the worst thing he can do to his feet). Then the degenerative arthritic process kicks in at a much faster rate—and the patient is much more likely to be forced into inactivity than he would have been had he simply cut down a little in the first place.

If you have arthritis in your ankles or feet, stretching exercises for the plantar fascia ligament and Achilles tendon are especially important. As you recall, arthritis is an inflammation of the cartilage in the joints—and cartilage is the body's prime shock absorber. So it's even more important to keep the other soft tissues flexible to make up for the wear and tear within the joints.

I'm exercising for the first time in my life as part of a weight-loss program, and it's working. But my feet feel absolutely terrible. How can I stop my sore feet from ruining the progress I'm making?

This is not an uncommon experience, and I know it's frustrating. You're told you need to exercise to lose weight, but as soon as you're beginning to enjoy and get results from your new diet-exercise regimen, your feet protest. Part of the problem is that walking is generally recommended as the ideal exercise—which it is!—at the beginning of a weight-loss program. However, it's important to realize that your feet probably aren't in the best shape right now, not only because they've been carrying around the extra weight for years but also because they're not accustomed to vigorous activity.

The stretches I recommended in this chapter should help you considerably, and you should always do them before beginning your daily exercise routine. If you're substantially overweight, however, that may not be enough. The heavier you are, the more likely you are to have developed sagging arches over the years. Orthotic inserts may well put an end to your pain during exercise. You should see a podiatrist and follow his or her recommendations for either over-the-counter or custom-made orthotics.

I once had a dramatic experience with a patient who, at 375 pounds, was actually in a life-threatening situation because of her weight. Marilyn was so desperate to lose weight that she'd gone on the phen-fen diet and lost 150 pounds. She was shifted to another, safer drug when phen-fen was withdrawn from the market after it was linked to fatal cardiac valve problems. By the time I saw her, Marilyn had regained most of the weight she had lost on phen-fen. Her arches were so flat (and her ankles so swollen) that she couldn't walk even one block. In her fifties, Marilyn worked behind the scenes at a high-tech company (because of her weight, no one would hire her for jobs dealing with the public), and she was having a difficult time just getting to her office. It's no exaggeration to say that she was desperate.

Marilyn had never been examined by a podiatrist, even though she had tried and failed to carry through with numerous exercise programs. I strapped her tightly and then cast her feet for a special heavy-duty pair of orthotics. I also advised her to wear a one-inch heel, as she'd been shuffling around in bedroom slippers that she mistakenly thought were right for her flat feet.

The results have been nothing less than remarkable, given where Marilyn started. This was a woman who, in her entire adult life, had never been able to walk more than a block. Now she's increased her daily walk to twelve blocks—and she's shooting for a mile a day. She is also losing five pounds a week, which could be a lifesaver for her. I can't predict the outcome of Marilyn's case at this point, but this is the first time she has ever successfully managed to combine diet with exercise. To see her walk out of my office in fitness shoes, preparing for a twenty-minute walk, instead of shuffling and wheezing into a taxi, is to feel hope for her. More important, she's feeling hopeful about herself. And that wouldn't be possible if we hadn't been able to do something about her feet.

Obviously, Marilyn's is an extreme case. But if you're trying to lose any significant amount—around 20 percent of your body weight—a podiatric consultation may help you stay on the right exercise track. Your body isn't used to the demands you're making on it, and your feet can use every bit of biomechanical help you can get. As you continue to lose weight, your feet will feel better and better, and your orthotics can be adjusted to fit your changing body.

I've just started walking and my feet feel fine, but I've suddenly developed lower back pain. Could my new exercise routine be the cause?

Yes. If you've recently had a physical (during the past three months), you can probably be confident that your back pain isn't caused by a systemic disease or serious disk problem. Insufficient arch support in walking shoes is one of the chief causes of back and foot pain in people who've recently begun to walk for fitness. You should consult a podiatrist and bring your fitness shoes along for an evaluation. You could have an extremely high arch, which lessens the ability of the foot to absorb the shock of each step. Or you may have fallen arches, which can place extra pressure on the lower back muscles because they're trying to compensate for the excessive weight shift toward the ball of your foot. The podiatrist will take a close look at your walking shoes (they may be designed with a weight shift that throws you further off balance) and recommend a different style. She may also prescribe a custom-made orthotic for your exercise shoes.

A podiatrist might also send you to a physical therapist to

learn special exercises designed to strengthen your abdominal muscles and stretch your lower back. If you have a history of back problems, you should be doing these exercises already. But don't use lower back pain as an excuse to return to your former level of inactivity. In nearly every case, I find that a change of shoes, coupled with use of orthotics, enables patients to return to walking without suffering from lower back pain. In fact, walking is an important component of exercise routines designed specifically to ameliorate back pain.

I've seen people walking with wrist and ankle weights, and I want to to increase the difficulty of my walking workouts. Is this likely to hurt me in any way?

I'd advise against it. I'm not opposed to working out with weights in a gym, but weights may place undue strain on your feet, ankles, knees, and lower back if you use them while you're walking. Think about it: A five-pound weight on each ankle places fifteen extra pounds of pressure on your feet. If your bones and joints can't stand up under the added pressure (and remember, the ankle is one of the most delicate and complex joints in your body), you'll have to cut back on walking in order to recover—and that will defeat your purpose in using weights in the first place. If you want to increase the difficulty of a walking workout, do it by slowly increasing the distance and your pace. If you're over thirty and want to work out with weights, start under the supervision of an experienced physical therapist or fitness trainer.

I recently had a bone density test, and I was upset to discover that I've lost a significant amount of bone mass since I entered menopause. My doctor advised me to begin a program of weight-bearing exercise, but I'm not really clear about what that involves. Why can't I just go on riding my exercise bike, which I do while I'm reading the paper?

Many people are confused by the term "weight-bearing exercise," because they think it has something to do with lifting weights. As I've already said, weight-bearing exercise means any activity that produces a direct impact between your foot and the ground, forcing your bones to bear the pressure of your body. Walking, jogging, dancing, and step aerobics are all weight-bearing exercises. Swimming and cycling are not, because your feet aren't supporting the weight of your body. Non-weight-bearing exercise has cardiovascular and other health benefits, but it won't help preserve your bone mass. Working out on StairMasters and treadmills has some weight-bearing value, but not as much as walking because the mechanical assistance reduces the impact.

Weight-bearing exercise will not restore the bone you've already lost, but, in combination with calcium (and hormone replacement or other drug therapies), it may help you preserve the bone you have and slow the rate of bone loss in the future. When you walk, as much as four hundred pounds of force travel up your legs and spine with every step. When you consider that you take seventy steps a minute if you walk a mile in a half hour (a slow pace for most exercisers), you can understand how much of a workout walking gives your bones. Your muscles tug on your bones, and this stimulates the bones to absorb more calcium.

I firmly believe that the dreaded dowager's hump—the worst manifestation of severe osteoporosis in previous generations of women—will one day become a thing of the past. For women in midlife, weight-bearing activity is one way to banish the fairy-tale specter of the humpbacked witch.

I live in a cold climate, and my feet often feel numb when I return home from my fitness walk during the winter. Should I be concerned?

If the sensation in your feet quickly returns once you're in a warm room, there's nothing to worry about. You just need to wear warmer socks. If the numbness persists for more than a few minutes, it's possible (though not likely) that you're in the early stages of frostbite. Don't place extremely chilled skin under hot water, because you might not realize that you're burning yourself. Heat up your cold feet slowly with lukewarm water.

You should see your doctor immediately if there has been a recent change in the reaction of your feet to the cold. Numbness in the feet is, as I've mentioned elsewhere in this book, one symptom of systemic diseases like diabetes. Any change in your usual responses to heat or cold could be cause for concern.

I used to love walking, but I'm getting bored with it. How can I get back the thrill? (Don't tell me to try another form of exercise, because bikes and treadmills are even more boring.) And my doctor says running would be too strenuous.

Ah, yes. The walker's slump. You used to feel proud of yourself for just getting out of the house. You smiled and nodded at the other walkers, pleased with yourself to be in such energetic company. You felt proud when you passed a slowpoke and competitive when you saw someone faster. You set goals for yourself. By the next month, you were walking a mile in fifteen minutes instead of twenty minutes. Now you're walking as fast as you can, and you can't think of any new goals to set. Your daily exercise has become just another chore.

The first thing you need to do is remind yourself why you started walking in the first place. Chances are that you were overweight, out of breath, or suffering from a multitude of middle-aged health problems (from high blood pressure to constipation) that your doctor told you could be helped by exercise. You've probably started to take the health benefits of walking for granted, which increases the temptation to stop.

You need to play some psychological games with yourself to revive your motivation.

One way to renew your interest is to change the geography of your walks. I know this isn't always easy, especially if you live in a cold climate and must walk indoors (usually in a gym or shopping mall) in winter. In temperate months, though, look for pleasant open spaces—some of them may be only a short drive from your home—that you haven't tried before. If you're worried about safety, call a local walkers' or runners' organization and find out where and when the real fitness fanatics train. You may find that dozens of exercisers gather every morning in a secluded local park, and you can tag along for the scenery. One man I know discovered that his local high school track team trained every spring morning along a river walk that he'd considered too isolated for safety. The students enjoyed his company (though they couldn't believe it when he turned down their proffered doughnuts at the end of his walk), and the gentle competition helped him step up his walking pace.

If you're in good health, you may also want to plan more challenging walks in real countryside. Check with your doctor if you're planning a walk that includes hills. Training for a walk in more rugged country can make your daily routine more challenging.

Another way to keep yourself on your feet is to promise yourself a small reward at the end of every week of walking. I call this the "bribe yourself" fitness plan. Buy yourself that new hardcover mystery novel instead of waiting patiently for it to come out in paperback. End your walk with a movie you've been dying to see. (This works only if you're a late-afternoon walker.) Purchase and prepare the foods you most love for breakfast and set everything out so that it will be waiting for you when you get home from your early-morning walk.

Many people (I'm not one of them) also enjoy listening to music or books on tape when they walk. I try to empty my mind and just enjoy the scenery in Central Park, because sometimes my best ideas surface when I'm concentrating on nothing but putting one foot in front of the other.

Another point: There may be people in your life who are discouraging you from walking, or at least encouraging you to "skip it just this once." This may be the time to seek reinforcement from like-minded exercisers who share your fitness goals. It's just as hard to reestablish the habit of walking as it is to start walking in the first place. Maybe even harder, because a return to the sedentary life has something of the depressing psychological impact of a drug or alcohol relapse.

I've lived with bunions and hammertoes for years, and they never caused me any real problems until I began exercising. Is there anything I can do short of surgery to enable me to continue my exercise program?

That's a tough one. Patients facing this dilemma are usually in their forties or fifties, and—as the question implies—they managed to live quite comfortably with bony foot deformities as long as they were sedentary. The problem is that severely damaged joints, even with the help of good fitness shoes and orthotics, often fail to hold up under the added pressure of weight-bearing exercise.

I'm assuming that you've already tried out various shoes and orthotics under the supervision of a podiatrist and a skilled pedorthist (a specialist in corrective shoe inserts) and nothing has helped. At this point, you will probably have to decide whether continuing your new active lifestyle is more important to you than avoiding surgery.

If you're in good general health and have been told by a doctor you respect that there's a good chance of correcting your long-standing bone deformities, I'd go ahead with an operation. One important factor to consider is whether you're likely to need surgery at a later date even if you put it off now. If you're fifty years old and have a bunion so painful that it won't stand up under a moderate fitness routine, the degeneration is likely to continue even if you stop exercising right now. (Remember, bunions are connected with arthritic changes.) Then you'll be facing bunion surgery at sixty in order to continue walking at all—and you'll have lost out on ten years of health-enhancing activity. I believe that surgery is the smart decision for otherwise healthy adults facing a choice between severe foot pain and a life without free movement.

29

How to Find the Best Medical Care for Your Lifestyle

There's a great deal of confusion about medical foot care, because two groups of professionals—podiatrists and orthopedists—are involved in the treatment of painful problems affecting feet and ankles. Orthopedists and podiatrists tend to view each other as professional competitors, and too many of them denigrate each other's skills to prospective patients. In public forums, many orthopedists act as if podiatrists don't exist, and vice versa. This is consumer-unfriendly nonsense, and I'll try to sort it out for you.

I'm a doctor of podiatric medicine (D.P.M.), which means that I spent four years at a podiatric medical school, followed by two years of surgical training in a special rotating surgical residency at several New York hospitals. I received additional postgraduate training at the New York University School of Medicine. Orthopedists are medical doctors (M.D.s), which means that they spent four years in medical school, followed by a year's hospital internship and a hospital residency of at least three years. It's fair to say that orthopedic surgeons have broader general medical training, while podiatric surgeons have more training in the specific problems of feet. (Not all podiatrists or orthopedists are certified to perform surgery.)

Are you thoroughly confused? There is also a subgroup of orthopedists, members of the American Orthopaedic Foot and Ankle Society, who have specialized advanced training in foot and ankle surgery. The real difference, in my opinion, is not between podiatrists and orthopedists per se but between those who have specialized training in foot conditions and those who don't. If you need medical attention for your feet—whether you have garden-variety corns and calluses or you need surgery—you want and deserve a doctor who has considerable experience with your particular problem. "How many operations of this kind have you performed?" is, as I mentioned earlier, one of the most important questions every patient should ask a prospective surgeon. Moreover, the management of many foot conditions requires close cooperation between podiatric specialists and medical doctors.

I work with M.D. internists, rheumatologists, and vascular surgeons to treat patients who suffer from foot problems caused by systemic diseases like diabetes and rheumatoid arthritis. They refer patients to me, and I refer patients to them. That's the way it should be. Moreover, there are many instances in which I suspect that a patient's foot troubles may be secondary to another orthopedic problem—a severely degenerated disk in the lower back, for example. Of course I recommend an orthopedic consultation for that person! How can I treat a foot properly if the primary problem is the patient's lower back?

Whatever type of practitioner you choose to handle your foot care, here are some of the most important issues to consider.

WHAT YOU SHOULD KNOW ABOUT YOUR DOCTOR

■ Has your podiatrist completed a surgical residency, and is he or she board-certified to perform surgery? The three boards that certify podiatric surgeons are the American Board of Podiatric Surgeons, the American Board of Podiatric Orthopedists, and the American Board of Ambulatory Surgery. While most podiatric surgical residencies last two years, there's now a special three-year residency that trains podiatrists to perform complicated ankle surgeries.

If you're interviewing an orthopedist, make sure that he or she has received specialized training in foot and ankle surgery. If you have any doubts about your prospective surgeon's qualifications, contact the American Podiatric Medical Association (APMA) in Washington, D.C., or the American Orthopaedic Foot and Ankle Society in Seattle. These organizations can refer you to a board-certified surgeon in your area. For podiatric referrals, call the APMA at 1-800 FOOTCARE or visit the Web site at www.APMA.org.

■ Is your doctor affiliated with a respected local hospital? Of course, there are mediocre doctors who have hospital staff privileges, but the *absence* of a hospital affiliation is a red flag. Also, if you're undergoing ambulatory surgery in a doctor's office or clinic, you'll want hospital backup in case anything goes wrong.

■ Does your doctor regularly participate in programs designed to acquaint medical professionals with new procedures and instruments in diagnosis and surgery? Because technological advances have transformed every branch of medicine during the past twenty years, doctors need to place continuous emphasis on updating their knowledge and skills. We learn how to use these new surgical and diagnostic tools by attending seminars and observing pioneers in the field. I've been both a student and a teacher at dozens of these sessions during the past fifteen years, and your doctor should have done the same.

- Has your doctor published articles in professional journals? This is easy to check out on the Internet. There are many outstanding doctors who don't publish professionally, but publication is *one* indicator of a doctor's standing among his or her peers.

- If your doctor recommends surgery, is he or she comfortable with your desire to get a second opinion? A good doctor, whether podiatrist or orthopedist, welcomes second opinions. Unless you're in an emergency situation, there's no reason not to acquire more information. I'm especially gratified when a patient of mine, after consulting someone else, chooses to have me operate. That patient is sure to have more faith in me and in the outcome of her surgery. As a patient, I would walk out on any doctor who objected to my getting a second opinion.

- Is the doctor experienced in treating patients with a lifestyle similar to yours? This may be the most important issue in choosing a medical professional. Most of us select doctors as a result of personal recommendations from friends and colleagues—and that's often the best way to find high-quality medical practitioners. But the most useful recommendations tend to come from people with similar medical needs. The doctor who did wonders for a dedicated thirty-year-old runner after an Achilles tendon rupture isn't necessarily the best person to treat a fifty-year-old who has developed aching arches because she's gained thirty pounds in the last twelve months.

You should rely only on recommendations from someone you know well and respect. Patients sometimes choose a doctor because he's known to treat prominent members of the community. Whether a "celebrity" recommendation comes from a wealthy local businessman or someone you've seen on television, there's no reason to assume that a rich and/or famous figure knows more about how to choose a doctor than your mother does. (In fact, mothers generally come up with great medical references.)

A WORD ABOUT MONEY AND MANAGED CARE

We all know that managed care is having a profound effect on doctor-patient relationships. Some patients are limited to doctors within their managed care networks, while others have health insurance that allows them, for a higher premium, to choose an out-of-network doctor if they so desire. Before managed care, if you needed a foot doctor you would probably have asked your primary care physician for a recommendation. But you can't always rely on that today—even if you have the highest respect for your doctor—because most physicians within managed care networks are contractually forbidden to refer patients to doctors outside the network. Your doctor might know an excellent podiatric surgeon, but he or she can't refer you if that podiatrist doesn't practice within the net. So if you have an insurance plan allowing you to use both in- and out-of-network doctors, you'll have to do your own homework.

I do not belong to any managed care network, and I'm fortunate that most of my patients have the kind of health insurance that allows them to choose their own doctors. However, I do have patients who, although they're able to pay for routine care out-of-network, are forced to stay inside their managed care plan when they need surgery. If you're in this situation, ask your usual podiatrist to go over the foot specialists on your managed care list and see if he or she knows any of them. Medicine, even in large cities, can be a very small world: Sometimes I spot outstanding former students of mine on a managed care list.

Another problem for patients is that even when their insurance plans reimburse for "usual and customary" out-of-network fees, there's generally a gap between what the company regards as "customary" and what doctors in the area actually charge. Although your insurance company may refuse to tell you up front what's usual and customary, your podiatrist probably knows what proportion of his or her fee is generally reimbursed under your plan. If you know in advance what you're likely to be asked to pay out of pocket, you and your doctor may be able to come up with a suitable plan for repayment. The days when doctors and patients didn't have to discuss fees in advance are probably gone for good. Candor on both sides can go a long way toward preventing the least desirable result—an angry doctor with an unpaid bill and an angry patient asked to pay more than she anticipated.

Afterword

*It may not be natural for a man to walk on
two legs, but it was a noble invention.*

—Georg Christoph Lichtenberg

Stay on your feet and don't take them for granted. That's my
basic message, whether you're a twenty-five-year-old marathon
runner at your physical peak or an eighty-five-year-old mall
walker trying to go the distance in spite of creaky ankles and
knees. It's only natural that our feet, because of the pounding
they take over tens of thousands of miles, begin to remind us of
our age before the rest of our body lets us know that it too
could benefit from a tune-up. One thing is certain: Since
Americans are living longer than ever before, we need to keep
our feet in better shape for the lengthening road ahead. It's certainly possible (even likely, I would say) that this century will
see the development of artificial joints to replace worn-out toes
and ankles as effectively as such devices now substitute for
badly degenerated hips. But no synthetic body part, however
remarkable a product of human inventiveness, can ever serve us
with the unparalleled combination of strength, flexibility, and
sensitivity endowed upon us at birth by our own flesh and
blood.

A generation ago, foot care specialists saw the relief of pain as their primary task; maintaining mobility (especially in older patients) was an important but definitely secondary goal. Today, pain relief and the preservation of mobility are equally important. My patients—whether they're in their thirties or their seventies—aren't satisfied to stop hurting if an end to pain means an end to doing what they love.

That's why I've placed so much emphasis on self-care and exercise in this book. Wearing the right shoes, paying attention to minor hurts, and exercising regularly not only help you avoid serious injuries as a young adult but also pay dividends down the road. You want your feet to last as long as the rest of you. I can use all of the tools of modern medicine to ease pain and repair injuries, but only you can take charge of the day-in, day-out maintenance that truly makes your feet fit for life.

Appendix A:
Quick First-Aid Fixes

Most injuries—as well as flare-ups of chronic foot conditions—seem to occur at times and in places when medical attention is more than a phone call or a fifteen-minute drive away. If it's Saturday night or you're away for the weekend, here's what to do for some of the most common foot emergencies until you can see a doctor.

ACHILLES TENDON PULL

If you're a veteran exerciser and this has happened to you before, you know what to do: Get off your feet and ice the area. (If you've actually ruptured your Achilles tendon as opposed to straining it, the pain will be so great that you'll probably head straight for the emergency room.) But if you're new to exercise and haven't experienced a strained or partially torn tendon, you may not recognize a potentially serious injury.

The important thing to remember is that if you feel *any* persistent pain—however mild—running up the back of your ankle, stop what you're doing and head for the ice. Ice the area for fifteen minutes out of every hour, especially if there's also ankle swelling. Don't exercise again until you've seen a podiatrist or orthopedist. Most full Achilles tendon ruptures can be avoided if the sufferer does not try to push on through the warning pain.

ANKLE SPRAIN

This is probably the most common leisure-time injury. You're out dancing or running around on a tennis court, you twist your ankle, and within a few moments it starts to swell and you can't bear to put any weight on it. The first half day after the injury, apply ice for at least fifteen minutes out of every hour. Try to keep the foot elevated above heart level, and don't use heat (a common mistake). Even if the swelling starts to go down, you must seek medical attention as soon as possible. You need an X ray to rule out any broken bones. Over-the-counter anti-inflammatories may provide some pain relief.

ARCH OR HEEL PAIN

If you have a sudden, sharp pain in your arch or heel while you're exercising or when you step out of bed, don't fool around with it. Rest your foot and ice it until you can get medical attention. There can be a number of causes, but the main thing is that you not continue to put weight on the area.

BUNION BURSA SWELLING

Cool it with ice for fifteen minutes every four to six hours. Over-the-counter analgesics, taken as directed, may help. And of course, stay off your feet. If the swelling isn't down significantly in twenty-four hours, see your podiatrist.

CORN BURSA SWELLING

Ice the area as you would for a bunion, then soak your feet in a solution of Epsom salts and warm water. This usually isn't as painful as a sudden bunion flare-up.

SHARP OBJECT IN FOOT

If it's very small and you can see it near the surface of the skin, disinfect the area and very gently try to pry out the foreign body with a small, sharp instrument you've sterilized with disinfectant. (You can use a sewing needle if you're sure it's sterile. But be careful; I've had patients who dropped the needle and stepped on that too.) If it hurts too much when you probe around the edge, the object is probably embedded too deeply. In that case, don't place weight on the area and have a podiatrist remove the invader after numbing the spot with local anesthetic.

TOENAIL INFECTION OR SWELLING

Wash the area gently and soak it in an iodine solution. Apply a topical antibiotic cream. See a doctor if the area continues to hurt, because the infection can spread.

TORN-OFF TOENAIL

Anyone who's ever torn a toenail well down into the nail bed knows how excruciatingly painful this small injury can be. Clean the area very gently with soap and water or a disinfectant (if you can stand the pain), apply topical antibiotic ointment, and cover with sterile gauze. You should see a podiatrist, because if the remaining portion of the nail isn't trimmed neatly and cleaned (this will be done under local anesthetic), you could wind up with a bad infection.

BLEEDING WART

This can be scary, because the small capillaries trapped within warts can bleed profusely if they're traumatized. If you already know you have a wart, there's nothing to worry about. You just need to get the bleeding under control with a thick gauze bandage or a sterile sponge. Stay off the area and see your podiatrist as soon as possible. The wart will probably have to be removed.

Appendix B:
Exercises

Throughout this book, I have emphasized the need for daily exercises designed to stretch your calf muscles and Achilles tendon. They are often recommended as part of rehabilitation after foot or ankle surgery, but I think they're even more important for prevention of plantar fascia ligament and Achilles tendon strains, as well as ankle sprains. I suggest that my patients do some combination of these stretches for ten minutes, twice a day. For those who engage in vigorous high-impact exercise, stretches are ideal for warming up and cooling down.

While these exercises are generally beneficial for people of all ages and fitness levels, you should consult your doctor or a physical therapist before beginning any routine. If you've led a sedentary life, you may not be sure exactly how far to push yourself, even with simple exercises like these.

Another note of caution: Make sure, when doing exercises that call for the use of a chair or footstool, that you've taken precautions against skidding. Place the chair against a wall and use a footstool only if it is level and has skid-preventing rubber tips. (Stools manufactured with safety in mind also have a rubber grip on the standing surface. Decorative wooden stools, covered with ordinary fabric, should never be used for exercise.) You can also use a step, if it has a rise high enough to accommodate your stretch. Don't ever place a footstool on a rug unless the carpet is firmly weighted down to the floor. It's best to do these exercises barefoot or wearing only socks, but do not wear socks—which can cause you to slip—if you're stretching against the wall on a bare floor.

STANDING CALF STRETCH

Place one foot on a stable footstool or chair, with the other foot pointed slightly outward on the floor (position A). Keeping both heels down, lean forward over the stool until you feel

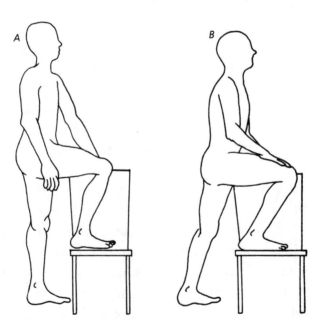

Figure 3. Standing calf stretch.

a stretching sensation in your calf (position B). Hold thirty seconds and repeat six times. Reverse foot positions and repeat on the other side.

STANDING DOUBLE CALF STRETCH

Stand about two feet away from a wall, with your feet together and pointed forward, your knees straight (position A). Place your palms (but not your full forearms) against the wall, lean your body forward, until you feel a stretching sensation in the back of the calf muscles (position B). *Make sure that your heels remain flat on the ground and you don't bend your back during this stretch.* Hold thirty seconds and repeat six times.

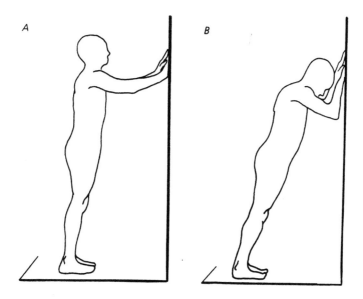

Figure 4. Standing double calf stretch.

DANGLING CALF STRETCH

Standing with both feet on a stable footstool or step, move one foot backward so that the hindfoot and heel hang over the edge (position A). Push the heel of the dangling foot down below the level of the stool or step, until you begin to feel a stretch in the calf muscles (position B). To increase the stretch, bend the other leg at the knee. Repeat three times and hold for thirty seconds. Reverse positions and repeat on the other side.

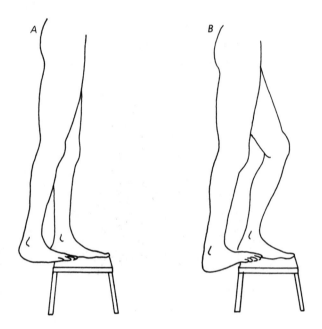

Figure 5. Dangling calf stretch.

STANDING CALF STRETCH (VARIATION)

This exercise is a variation of the first standing calf stretch, and it doesn't require a chair or footstool. Stand with your front foot turned forward, about two feet from a wall, and with your back foot on the floor turned slightly outward. Bend forward leg slightly at the knee, keeping the back leg straight. Bracing yourself against the wall with your hands, lean forward until you feel a stretch in the calf of the forward leg—keeping the heel of the back leg firmly down on the floor. Hold thirty seconds and repeat six times. Reverse positions and repeat.

PLANTAR FASCIA LIGAMENT STRETCH

Sit on an ordinary chair and hoist one leg up over the other, with your ankle resting on your opposite knee. Grasp your toes and pull them *gently* backward, until you feel a stretch in the arch of your foot. Hold thirty seconds and repeat six times with each foot.

For a quick fix if you wake up with arch pain, try sitting on a couch and putting your legs on a coffee table. Place a long muffler-type scarf under the ball of your foot. Holding the ends of the scarf, pull them gently toward you until you feel a stretch in the arch. Hold thirty seconds and repeat six times. However, discontinue this exercise if your pain intensifies.

Index

accidents to feet, 213–16
Achilles tendinitis, 108, 113–21, 207, 233
Achilles tendon (heel cord), 4, 8–11
 avoiding injuries to, 261
 exercise for, 81, 93, 112, 119, 239
 first-aid for, 257–58
 injuries to, 113–21, 257–58
 painful, in the morning, 91
 rupture of, 79–80
 shoes that reduce strain on, 185
 shortened, from high heels, 83, 181
 tightness of, 74, 90, 110
Acumassage, 220
acupuncture, 220, 225
adolescents. *See* teens
adult-onset diabetes, 148
aerobic exercise, 234, 243
African Americans
 and corns, 171–72
 and foot problems, 22–23
 and skin discoloration, 162, 171–72
aged. *See* elderly
aging
 and increase in shoe size, 21–22
 normal process of, 204
AIDS, 165
alcohol, as remedy, 44, 70
alignment of bones, 153
allergies, 40, 216

alternative medical care, 222–28
American Board of Ambulatory Surgery, 250
American Board of Podiatric Orthopedists, 250
American Board of Podiatric Surgeons, 250
American Orthopaedic Foot and Ankle Society (AOFAS), 30, 249, 250
American Podiatric Medical Association (APMA), 250
American Society of Plastic and Reconstructive Surgeons, 171
anesthesia, types of, 134–35, 228
ankle
 fat, 174–75
 osteoporosis of, 206–7
 sprained, 108–9, 111–12, 116
  avoiding, 261
  first-aid for, 258
  swollen, 143, 193–94
ankle block (anesthesia), 135
ankle bone (talus), 8
ankle joint (subtalus), 4, 8
ankle weights, to be avoided, 242
antalgic gait, 12, 91
antibacterial cream, 41
antibiotics, 42
 during pregnancy, 194–95
antidepressants, for pain, 228

About the Author

S UZANNE M. L EVINE, D.P.M., a podiatric surgeon in private practice in Manhattan for twenty years, has been a pioneer in ambulatory, in-office foot surgery. She is a clinical podiatrist and supervisor of podiatric interns at New York Presbyterian-Cornell Medical Center, and she is also on staff at Manhattan Eye, Ear, and Throat Hospital. Dr. Levine, who received her Doctor of Podiatric Medicine Degree from the New York College of Podiatric Medicine and a master's degree in physical therapy from Columbia University, has achieved recognition in what is still a male-dominated profession. Only 8 percent of podiatric surgeons are women.

The author of *My Feet Are Killing Me!* (1986), *Walk It Off* (1992), and *50 Ways to Ease Foot Pain* (1993), Dr. Levine speaks frequently to corporate and consumer audiences on health issues. Her corporate clients have included Revlon, Merrill Lynch, and American Express. She has also served as a medical consultant for manufacturers of walking shoes.

Dr. Levine is a board-certified podiatric surgeon (Ambulatory Division, American Board of Foot Surgeons) and a member of the American Society for Laser Medicine Surgery. Her Web site is www.institutebeaute.com.

6 6-7
40
645
166/167
168/169